Handbook of Multiple Sclerosis

Second edition

Handbook of Multiple Sclerosis

Second edition

Jeffrey A Cohen, MD
Alexander Rae-Grant, MD, FRCP(C)
Mellen Center for Multiple Sclerosis Treatment and Research
Neurologic Institute
Cleveland Clinic Foundation
Cleveland, OH

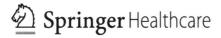

Springer Healthcare

Published by Springer Healthcare Ltd, 236 Gray's Inn Road, London, WC1X 8HB, UK.

www.springerhealthcare.com

© 2012 Springer Healthcare, a part of Springer Science+Business Media.

First edition 2010
Revised edition 2012

British Library Cataloguing-in-Publication Data.

A catalogue record for this book is available from the British Library.

ISBN 978-1-908517-49-4

Although every effort has been made to ensure that drug doses and other information are presented accurately in this publication, the ultimate responsibility rests with the prescribing physician. Neither the publisher nor the authors can be held responsible for errors or for any consequences arising from the use of the information contained herein. Any product mentioned in this publication should be used in accordance with the prescribing information prepared by the manufacturers. No claims or endorsements are made for any drug or compound at present under clinical investigation.

Project editor: Tess Salazar
Designer: Joe Harvey
Artworker: Sissan Mollerfors
Production: Marina Maher
Printed in the UK by Latimer Trend and Co. Ltd.

Contents

	Author biographies	vii
	Abbreviations	ix
1	**Introduction**	**1**
	Pathology and pathogenesis	1
	Genetics	4
	Epidemiology	5
	References	6
2	**Clinical features**	**7**
	Clinical manifestations	7
	Course	7
	Prognosis	12
	References	13
3	**Diagnosing multiple sclerosis**	**15**
	Investigations	15
	Diagnostic criteria	19
	Differential diagnosis	22
	References	27
4	**Treatment of acute relapses of multiple sclerosis**	**29**
	References	32
5	**Disease-modifying therapy**	**35**
	Disease-modifying agents	35
	Initiating, monitoring, and changing therapy in relapsing–remitting multiple sclerosis	44
	Clinically isolated syndromes	47
	Treatment of progressive multiple sclerosis	48
	Treatment of fulminant multiple sclerosis	49
	Multiple sclerosis treatment in children	49
	Devic's neuromyelitis optica	50

Emerging anti-inflammatory therapies   51

References   55

6 Symptom management   **61**

General points   61

Impaired mobility   61

Diplopia and oscillopsia   68

Vertigo   68

Bulbar dysfunction   69

Spasticity   69

Tremor   71

Bladder dysfunction   71

Bowel dysfunction   74

Sexual dysfunction   74

Cognitive impairment   75

Mood disorders   76

Fatigue   77

Positive sensory phenomena and pain   78

References   80

**7 Medical management of patients with
multiple sclerosis**   **83**

Health maintenance   83

Immunizations   83

Sleep   84

Smoking   84

Reproductive health   84

Multidisciplinary care   85

References   85

Resources   **87**

Books   87

General information and best practices   87

Information on clinical trials   87

References   88

Author biographies

Jeffrey A Cohen, MD, is Professor of Medicine (Neurology) in the Cleveland Clinic Lerner College of Medicine of Case Western Reserve University and has worked at the Cleveland Clinic's Mellen Center for Multiple Sclerosis Treatment and Research since 1994. Dr Cohen received his BA in Zoology from Connecticut College in 1976 and MD from the University of Chicago Pritzker School of Medicine in 1980. He completed a neurology residency in 1984, then a 3-year neuroimmunology fellowship with Robert Lisak, MD, and Mark Greene, MD, at the University of Pennsylvania. He was on the faculty in the department of neurology at the University of Pennsylvania from 1987 to 1994. Dr Cohen's research interests included autoimmune mechanisms, antiviral immunity, lymphocyte activation, and glial biology as they relate to multiple sclerosis (MS). Dr Cohen moved to the Cleveland Clinic in 1994 to direct the Mellen Center's Experimental Therapeutics Program. He has been involved in various capacities in a large number of clinical trials developing new therapies for MS. In addition, he has helped develop new clinical and imaging endpoints for MS trials. At the Mellen Center, Dr Cohen also directs the Clinical Neuroimmunology Fellowship that has trained a number of MS clinical investigators. Finally, Dr Cohen has a large clinical practice devoted to the diagnosis and management of MS and related disorders.

Alexander Rae-Grant, MD, FRCP(C), is a staff neurologist at the Cleveland Clinic. He holds the Jane and Lee Seidman Chair for Advanced Neurological Education at the Cleveland Clinic. After receiving his Bachelor of Arts in biochemistry and molecular biology from Yale in 1979, he graduated from McMaster University Medical School in 1982. He completed 2 years of internal medicine at the University of Toronto followed by a neurology residency at the University of Western Ontario in 1987. Dr Rae-Grant joined the Cleveland Clinic's Mellen Center for Multiple Sclerosis Treatment and Research in 2007, where he is engaged in patient care and clinical trials and directs the patient and professional educational efforts. He is active in medical student, resident, and fellow training and co-directs the neurosciences clinical clerkship in the Cleveland Clinic Lerner College of Medicine. Dr Rae-Grant was recently honored as "Teacher of the year" for the Neurology Department at the Cleveland Clinic. He authored the neurology textbook *Neurology for the House Officer* and co-edited *The 5-Minute Consult in Neurology.*

Abbreviations

ALT	alanine transaminase
ANA	antinuclear antibodies
AST	aspartate transaminase
CBC	complete blood count
CC	corpus callosum
CIS	clinically isolated syndrome
CMP	comprehensive metabolic panel
CN	Canada
CNS	central nervous system
CSF	cerebrospinal fluid
CSO	centrum semiovale
DIS	dissemination in space
DIT	dissemination in time
EDSS	Expanded Disability Status Scale
EU	European Union
FDA	US Food and Drug Administration
Gd	gadolinium
GWAS	genome-wide association studies
IFN-β	interferon-beta
IgG	immunoglobulin G
LV	lateral ventricle
MHC	major histocompatibility complex
MRI	magnetic resonance imaging
MS	multiple sclerosis
MSWS-12	12-item Multiple Sclerosis Walking Scale
NAb	neutralizing antibody
NMO	neuromyelitis optica
PML	progressive multifocal leukoencephalopathy
PP	primary progressive
QOL	quality of life
RR	relapsing–remitting

S1P1	sphingosine-1-phosphate receptor 1
SP	secondary progressive
T25FW	Timed 25-Foot Walk
TOUCH	Tysabri Outreach: Unified Commitment to Health
TSH	thyroid-stimulating hormone
USA	United States of America

Chapter 1

Introduction

Multiple sclerosis (MS) is a chronic inflammatory disease of the central nervous system (CNS) that produces demyelination and axonal/neuronal damage, resulting in characteristic multifocal lesions on magnetic resonance imaging (MRI) and a variety of neurologic manifestations (Figure 1.1). The clinical manifestations typically first develop in young adults as acute relapses, and then evolve into a gradually progressive course with permanent disability after 10–15 years. It is important to make the diagnosis of MS accurately and expeditiously to relieve uncertainty and allow the institution of disease-modifying therapy. The purpose of therapy is to decrease relapses and MRI activity, with the ultimate goal of reducing the long-term risk of permanent disability. Furthermore, because of the myriad of potential manifestations that interfere with function and negatively impact quality of life (QOL), symptom management also is an important aspect of management.

Pathology and pathogenesis

The pathology of MS is characterized by multifocal lesions within the CNS, both in the white matter and gray matter (Figure 1.2), with perivenular inflammatory cell infiltrates, demyelination, axonal transection, neuronal degeneration, and gliosis (Figure 1.3) [1].

The pathogenesis of MS is complex and multifactorial [2]. Emerging concepts concerning the pathogenesis of MS are summarized in Figure 1.4. Traditional theory postulates that myelin-specific CD4+ T cells play a

J. A. Cohen and A. Rae-Grant, *Handbook of Multiple Sclerosis*,
DOI: 10.1007/978-1-907673-50-4_1, © Springer Healthcare 2012

Key clinical features of MS

Typical onset is in the age range 20–40 years

Female predominance ~2.5:1

Neurologic manifestations reflect multifocal involvement of the CNS (brain, spinal cord, optic nerves)

Nonfocal manifestations (eg, cognitive impairment, mood disorders, pain, and fatigue) also significantly contribute to disability

Relapsing–remitting course at onset in 70–80% of patients, usually evolving into a secondary progressive phase

Progressive course from onset in ~20% of patients

Most patients develop disability over 10–15 years

The range and severity of clinical manifestations have marked heterogeneity, both in individual patients over time and between patients

Diagnosis is straightforward in typical patients, but differential diagnosis is extensive when there are atypical features

Effective therapies are available and should be considered early to lessen the risk of permanent disability

Treatment of symptoms and addressing psychosocial sequelae are important aspects of management

Figure 1.1 Key clinical features of MS. CNS, central nervous system.

Pathology of MS

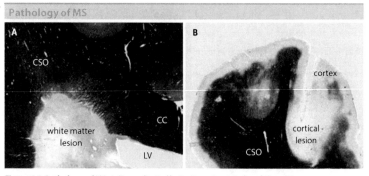

Figure 1.2 Pathology of MS. A, Demyelinated lesion in periventricular white matter;
B, Demyelinated lesion in cortex. CSO, centrum semiovale; CC, corpus callosum; LV, lateral ventricle.

central role in MS pathogenesis. Other T cell subsets, natural killer cells, monocytes/macrophages, B cells (both as producers of antibody and antigen-presenting cells), and humoral factors have been implicated.

In addition, studies of a large number of biopsy and autopsy specimens suggested that the mechanisms leading to tissue damage differ from patient to patient [3]. Ongoing studies are investigating the relationship

High-power view of a white matter lesion in MS

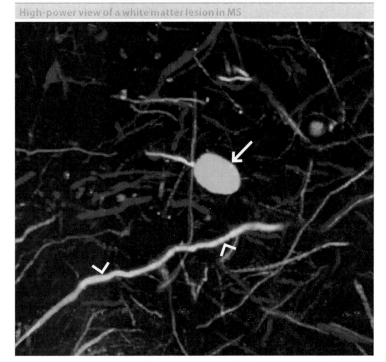

Figure 1.3 High-power view of a white matter lesion in MS. This confocal micrograph shows demyelination (arrowheads) and axonal transection (arrow).

Emerging concepts in pathogenesis of MS

MRI studies demonstrate ongoing subclinical disease activity

Pathology includes both demyelination and axonal damage, in both white and gray matter

Pathogenesis is complex, including both T and B cell mechanisms

Pathogenesis is heterogeneous, varying from patient to patient

Pathogenesis is inflammatory early, and degenerative late and in purely progressive MS

Compensatory mechanisms, repair and plasticity, are active early but fail late

The underlying etiology remains unknown

Recent data have shown that cortical lesions are common and may be an early feature of MS pathology

Leptomeningeal inflammatory nodules have been noted as a feature of MS pathology

Figure 1.4 Emerging concepts in pathogenesis of MS.

between pathogenic patterns, clinical and imaging characteristics, and response to therapy.

Finally, it appears that inflammatory mechanisms predominate early in the disease (reflected most directly in clinical relapses and MRI lesion activity), but the gradual worsening in primary progressive (PP) MS and late in the disease in secondary progressive (SP) MS are due to neurodegeneration [4]. Intrinsic repair mechanisms function in MS and are effective early but, in most patients, over time they become insufficient to compensate for ongoing damage, resulting in accrual of permanent disability. For example, oligodendrocyte precursors can be demonstrated in chronic lesions but appear unable to remyelinate dystrophic axons [5]. An important implication of these observations is that therapeutic strategies need to address multiple pathogenic mechanisms.

Genetics

Relatives of patients with MS are at increased risk for the disease (Figure 1.5), and several lines of evidence (Figure 1.6) indicate that MS has a genetic component [6,7]. However, the genetic basis of MS is complex (ie, multiple genes contribute cumulatively to the risk of MS and disease behavior) and is heterogeneous (ie, the genes and alleles involved probably differ from patient to patient). Genetic studies have most consistently implicated genes encoded in the class II region of the major histocompatibility complex (MHC) on chromosome 6, specifically the HLA-DR2 haplotype DRB1*1501-DQB1*0602 [8]. It is postulated that the MHC–disease association results from effects on antigen-presenting

Population-based prevalence of MS in relatives of patients with MS	
Cohort	**Prevalence (per 1000)**
General population	1
Adopted siblings	1
First cousin	7
Sibling	35
Child	197
Offspring of conjugal MS pair	200
Monozygotic twin	270

Figure 1.5 Population-based prevalence of MS in relatives of patients with MS.
Adapted from Ebers [7].

Evidence that MS has genetic aspects
MS is relatively common in people of Northern European descent and rare in Asians, Native Americans, and Gypsies
The risk of MS is increased 20- to 30-fold in first-degree relatives and up to 500-fold in monozygotic twins
Dizygotic twins have the same risk as siblings
Adoptees and spouses have the same risk as unrelated individuals
Genetic studies have implicated several loci, particularly the HLA-DR2 haplotype DRB1*1501-DQB1*0602

Figure 1.6 Evidence that MS has genetic aspects. Adapted from Ebers [7].

cells, altering immune reactivity to auto-antigens (possibly myelin-related auto-antigens).

Recent advances in genotyping platforms and the development of more effective statistical methods have resulted in the identification of more than 20 additional susceptibility loci by genome-wide association studies (GWAS), including genes encoding components of the interleukin-2 and interleukin-7 receptors [9]. These additional MS susceptibility alleles exert modest individual effects on risk compared with MHC but confirm the likelihood that multiple separate (though possibly overlapping) genes determine the risk for developing MS and disease behavior [10]. A recent GWAS – the largest MS genetics study ever undertaken, involving nearly 10,000 cases and more than 17,000 controls – identified 29 new genetic variants associated with MS and confirmed 23 others previously associated with the disease [11]. Genes that influence T cell maturation were significantly overrepresented among those mapping close to the identified loci, verifying a major role for the immune system in the pathogenesis of MS.

Epidemiology

The prevalence of MS is approximately 1/1000, affecting approximately 400,000 people in the USA and 2 million worldwide [12]. It is the most common nontraumatic cause of neurologic disability in young adults. Onset typically is between the ages of 20 and 40 years, and women are affected more frequently than men (approximately 2.5:1).

Approximately 70% of monozygotic twins are discordant for MS (ie, more than half of the monozygotic twins of patients with MS do not develop MS). This observation implies there is an interaction between the genetic propensity for MS and environmental factors. Epidemiologic studies demonstrated unequal geographic distribution of MS. There is a distinct latitude gradient: MS is relatively rare in the tropics and increases in prevalence with increasing latitude in both the northern and southern hemispheres. Migration studies suggest that the risk of acquiring MS is determined at the time of puberty or before. Postulated factors include infectious agents, diet, environmental toxins, and sunlight [7], but none has been definitively implicated.

References

1 Lucchinetti CF, Parisi J, Bruck W. The pathology of multiple sclerosis. *Neurol Clin.* 2005;23:77-105.

2 Frohman EM, Racke MK, Raine CS. Multiple sclerosis – the plaque and its pathogenesis. *N Engl J Med.* 2006;354:942-955.

3 Morales Y, Parisi JE, Lucchinetti CF. The pathology of multiple sclerosis: evidence for heterogeneity. *Adv Neurol.* 2006;98:27-45.

4 Trapp BD, Nave K-A. Multiple sclerosis: an immune or neurodegenerative disorder? *Annu Rev Neurosci.* 2008;31:247-269.

5 Chang A, Tourtellotte WW, Rudick RA, et al. Premyelinating oligodendrocytes in chronic lesions of multiple sclerosis. *N Engl J Med.* 2002;346:165-173.

6 Dyment DA, Ebers GC, Sadovnick AD. Genetics of multiple sclerosis. *Lancet Neurol.* 2004;3:104-110.

7 Ebers GC. Environmental factors and multiple sclerosis. *Lancet Neurol.* 2008;7:268-277.

8 The International Multiple Sclerosis Genetics Consortium. A high-density screen for linkage in multiple sclerosis. *Am J Hum Genet.* 2005;77:454-467.

9 The International Multiple Sclerosis Genetics Consortium. Risk alleles for multiple sclerosis identified by a genomewide study. *N Engl J Med.* 2007;357:851-862.

10 Hensiek AE, Seaman SR, Barcellos LF, et al. Familial effects on the clinical course of multiple sclerosis. *Neurology.* 2007;68:376-383.

11 The International Multiple Sclerosis Genetics Consortium & the Welcome Trust Case Control Consortium. Genetic risk and a primary role for cell-mediated immune mechanisms in multiple sclerosis. *Nature.* 2011;476:214-219.

12 Marrie RA. Environmental risk factors in multiple sclerosis aetiology. *Lancet Neurol.* 2004;3:709-718.

Chapter 2

Clinical features

Clinical manifestations

The wide range of symptoms and signs of multiple sclerosis (MS) reflect multifocal lesions in the central nervous system (CNS), including in the afferent visual pathways, cerebrum, brainstem, cerebellum, and spinal cord (Figure 2.1). In general, the range and severity of manifestations in an individual at a particular time reflect the extent of lesions, their location, the severity of tissue damage, and the rate of accumulation. However, the correlation between lesions, as visualized on standard magnetic resonance imaging (MRI), and clinical manifestations is only approximate. This may be because repair and neural plasticity may compensate for damage and residual function may not parallel changes on MRI images. In addition, recent work showed there is pathology in both white and gray matter not visible on standard MRI. A number of MS manifestations are frequently underappreciated, including cognitive impairment, psychiatric disorders, pain, and fatigue, but often are major contributors to disability.

Course

As summarized in Figure 2.2, the course of MS is categorized based on how clinical manifestations develop over time and on the severity and tempo of the disease [1].

J. A. Cohen and A. Rae-Grant, *Handbook of Multiple Sclerosis*,
DOI: 10.1007/978-1-907673-50-4_2, © Springer Healthcare 2012

Typical clinical manifestations of MS

Category	Description
Vision	Visual loss – monocular (pre-chiasmatic) or homonymous (post-chiasmatic)
	Double vision
	Oscillopsia
Vestibular symptoms	Vertigo
	Imbalance
Bulbar dysfunction	Dysarthria
	Swallowing dysfunction
Motor	Weakness
	Spasticity
	Incoordination
	Tremor
Abnormalities of sensation	Sensory loss – any modality or distribution
	Positive sensory phenomena – paresthesias, dysesthesias, neuropathic pain
Gait impairment	Varying contributions from visual impairment, vestibular symptoms, weakness, spasticity, ataxia, imbalance, sensory loss, pain, and fatigue
Urinary symptoms	Urgency
	Frequency
	Hesitancy
	Retention
	Incontinence
	Frequent urinary tract infections
Bowel symptoms	Constipation
	Urgency
	Incontinence
Sexual dysfunction	Decreased libido
	Erectile dysfunction
	Anorgasmia
Cognitive impairment	Poor concentration or attention
	Slowed thinking
	Poor memory, particularly short-term
	Impaired executive function
Mood disorders	Depression
	Anxiety
	Affective release

Figure 2.1 Typical clinical manifestations of MS (continues opposite).

Category	Description
Fatigue	Handicap fatigue – increased effort to perform routine tasks
	Motor fatigue – decreased performance or endurance with sustained effort
	Heat intolerance – worsening sensory or motor symptoms/signs with increased body temperature
	Systemic fatigue – persistent lassitude
Pain	Chronic neuropathic pain, paresthesias, dysesthesias
	Paroxysmal sensory symptoms (eg, neuralgic pain, Lhermitte's phenomenon, pseudoradiculopathy)
	Spasticity (eg, spasms, uncomfortable increased muscle tone)
	Paroxysmal motor phenomena (eg, tonic spasms, paroxysmal dystonia)
	Pain associated with acute inflammatory lesions and irritation of adjacent meninges (eg, optic neuritis, transverse myelitis)
	Chronic photophobia following optic neuritis
	Bladder spasms
	Mechanical back or joint pain from immobility
	Compression fractures
Paroxysmal phenomena	Epileptic seizures
	Nonepileptic paroxysmal motor phenomena (eg, paroxysmal dystonia, hemifacial spasm)
	Nonepileptic paroxysmal sensory phenomena (eg, Lhermitte's phenomenon)
	Uthoff's phenomenon

Title: Typical clinical manifestations of MS (continued)

Figure 2.1 Typical clinical manifestations of MS (continued).

The typical course of MS is depicted in Figure 2.3. In 70–80% of patients MS begins with a relapsing–remitting (RR) course. A relapse (also known as an exacerbation or attack) [2,3] is defined as:

- new, worsening, or recurrent neurologic symptoms consistent with those caused by MS;
- typically developing over days to weeks;
- lasting at least 24–48 hours; and
- accompanied by an objective change on the neurologic examination corresponding to the patient's symptoms.

Even without treatment, most relapses recover partially or completely over weeks to months, particularly early in the disease. However, not all relapses recover completely, and early in the disease most impairment/disability accrual is the result of incomplete relapse recovery [4]. Relapses are heterogeneous within and between patients in terms of

Clinical categories of MS

Category	Description
Clinically isolated syndrome (CIS)	One episode of inflammatory CNS demyelination
	Patients with a CIS are at increased risk of developing RR MS if there are multiple additional lesions on MRI or evidence of intrathecal antibody production in CSF
Relapsing–remitting (RR) MS	Recurrent episodes of inflammatory CNS inflammation with stable clinical manifestations between episodes (the initial course in ~70–80% of patients)
Secondary progressive (SP) MS	Gradual neurologic deterioration, with or without superimposed relapses, in a patient with prior RR MS
Primary progressive (PP) MS	Gradual neurologic deterioration from onset without superimposed relapses (~15–20% of patients)
Progressive-relapsing MS	Gradual neurologic deterioration from onset with subsequent superimposed relapses (~5% of patients)
Fulminant	Severe MS with frequent relapses and/or rapid disability progression (~5% of patients)
Benign	MS that remains mild over a prolonged course with rare relapses and minimal disability accumulation (~10–20% of patients)

Figure 2.2 Clinical categories of MS. CNS, central nervous system; CSF, cerebrospinal fluid.

Typical disease course in relapsing MS

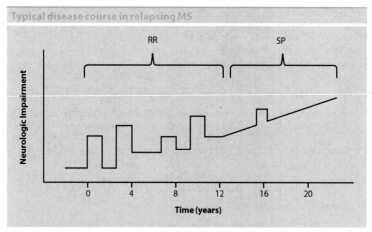

Figure 2.3 Typical disease course in relapsing MS. In 70–80% of patients, MS begins with a RR course. The initial relapse is a CIS. The diagnosis of RR MS is confirmed when a second clinical or MRI event occurs. In RR MS disability accrues from incomplete recovery from relapses. Relapses vary in neurologic manifestations, frequency, severity, and degree of recovery. Most patients with RR MS evolve into a SP course 10–15 years after onset. The transition from RR to SP MS is indistinct, with decreasing relapse frequency and onset of gradual worsening between relapses. Late in the disease, there is gradual progression without relapses. CIS, clinically isolated syndrome; RR, relapsing–remitting; SP, secondary progressive.

neurologic manifestations, frequency, severity, and degree of recovery. In practice, relapses may be indistinct or equivocal. Indeed, although a relapse is a clinical event, MS disease activity, as indicated by MRI lesion activity, can occur without clinical manifestations (ie, an MRI relapse). When a patient has had only a single relapse, the initial event is called a clinically isolated syndrome (CIS). The diagnosis of RR MS is confirmed when a recurrent CNS inflammatory event occurs, either a second relapse or new MRI lesion activity.

Patients with MS often experience worsening of pre-existing symptoms or reappearance of previous symptoms in the setting of infection or other intercurrent illness. These "pseudo-relapses" must be distinguished from bona fide relapses because they may indicate a condition that requires treatment and their ramification for long-term MS treatment differs. Acute relapses also must be distinguished from the transient fluctuations in manifestations that patients with MS frequently experience: transient worsening associated with increased body temperature (Uthoff's phenomenon), single paroxysmal symptoms (eg, Lhermitte's phenomenon or trigeminal neuralgia), or gradual worsening over months (ie, progression).

After 10–15 years most patients with RR MS exhibit gradual worsening of disability, known as the secondary progressive (SP) phase [5]. Sometimes there are continued superimposed relapses initially during the transition from RR to SP MS, but eventually there is continued progression in the absence of relapses and new MRI lesion activity.

Approximately 15% of patients with MS demonstrate gradual worsening disability from onset, known as have primary progressive (PP) MS. The clinical manifestations of PP MS frequently include a myelopathy (pyramidal manifestations in the legs and arms), or, less often, cerebellar, afferent visual, or cognitive symptoms. Patients with PP MS tend to be older at onset than those with relapsing forms of MS and there is less of a female predominance. A small proportion of patients with gradual worsening at onset experience subsequent superimposed relapses, called progressive-relapsing MS.

The biologic distinction between PP MS and relapsing forms of MS is not known. Similarly, the mechanisms that underlie the transition from RR to SP MS and gradual worsening in purely progressive MS (ie, late SP MS and PP MS) are poorly understood. It is thought that the accumulation of irreversible axonal damage and the possible development of a degenerative process are important.

Prognosis

As for other chronic diseases, severity varies among patients with MS. Decisions regarding treatment, career, and family planning are based on prognosis. Ultimately, however, it is difficult to make accurate prognostic predictions in individual patients early in the disease when these decisions need to be made. Approximately 5% of patients have fulminant MS with frequent relapses and/or rapid disability progression. Conversely, 10–20% of patients have benign MS that remains mild over a prolonged course with rare relapses and minimal disability accumulation. Clinicians must be careful not to prematurely reassure patients that they have benign disease early in the course or to miss disabling cognitive impairment in patients who have mild physical manifestations.

Several features are potentially prognostic of a good or bad course in MS and are listed in Figure 2.4. The presence of multiple MRI lesions at the time of CIS, and to a lesser extent intrathecal antibody production in the cerebrospinal fluid (CSF), indicate increased risk of subsequent clinical or MRI events that will lead to the diagnosis of RR MS [6].

Prognostic factors in MS	
Factors suggesting a more favorable prognosis	**Factors suggesting an unfavorable prognosis**
Female sex	Male sex
Predominantly sensory symptoms	Predominantly pyramidal, cerebellar, or cognitive symptoms
RR course	Progressive course
Infrequent, mild relapses with good recovery	Frequent, severe relapses with poor recovery
Prolonged time to onset of progressive course and/or accumulation of disability	Short time to onset of progressive course and/or accumulation of disability
Modest MRI lesions activity, mild T2-hyperintense and T1-hypointense lesion burden and atrophy, with slow MRI progression	Prominent and persistent MRI lesion activity, extensive T2-hyperintense and T1-hypointense lesion burden and atrophy, and rapid MRI progression

Figure 2.4 Prognostic factors in MS. RR, relapsing–remitting.

Furthermore, several features in the early course of MS predict overall prognosis in MS [7]. Nevertheless, although the presence of worrisome features often indicates poor prognosis, some patients show spontaneous improvement. More importantly, the absence of poor prognostic features may be misleading.

References

1   Lublin FD, Reingold SC. Defining the clinical course of multiple sclerosis: Results of an international survey. *Neurology.* 1996;46:907-911.

2   Schumacher GA, Beebe GW, Kibler RF, et al. Problems of experimental trials of therapy in multiple sclerosis: Report by the panel on the evaluation of experimental trials of therapy in multiple sclerosis. *Ann N Y Acad Sci.* 1965;122:552-568.

3   Polman CH, Reingold SC, Edan G, et al. Diagnostic criteria for multiple sclerosis: 2005 revisions to the "McDonald Criteria". *Ann Neurol.* 2005;58:840-846.

4   Lublin FD, Baier M, Cutter G. Effect of relapses on development of residual deficit in multiple sclerosis. *Neurology.* 2003;61:1528-1532.

5   Weinshenker BG, Bass B, Rice GPA, et al. The natural history of multiple sclerosis: A geographically based study. I. Clinical course and disability. *Brain.* 1989;112:133-146.

6   Brex PA, Ciccarelli O, O'Riordan JI, et al. A longitudinal study of abnormalities on MRI and disability from multiple sclerosis. *N Engl J Med.* 2002;346:158-164.

7   Weinshenker BG, Bass B, Rice GP, et al. The natural history of multiple sclerosis: a geographically based study. 2. Predictive value of the early clinical course. *Brain.* 1989;112:1419-1428.

Chapter 3

Diagnosing multiple sclerosis

Making an accurate and expeditious diagnosis of multiple sclerosis (MS) is important to allow the timely institution of disease-modifying therapy. Accurate diagnosis also removes uncertainty, and allows informed career and family planning. However, with the push to make the diagnosis early, there is increased risk of misdiagnosis.

Investigations

History

When a diagnosis of MS is being considered, the history should focus on:

- the range of neurologic symptoms;
- the time course over which the neurologic symptoms developed and improved;
- the effects of therapeutic interventions; and
- manifestations that suggest the presence of other conditions that could contribute to neurologic symptoms or indicate an MS mimic.

Physical examination

The physical examination focuses on assessing the presence of neurologic manifestations, specifically to determine whether they indicate a process with multifocal involvement of the central nervous system (CNS). Aspects of the general examination also may be useful if there are symptoms suggesting an alternative diagnosis.

J. A. Cohen and A. Rae-Grant, *Handbook of Multiple Sclerosis*,
DOI: 10.1007/978-1-907673-50-4_3, © Springer Healthcare 2012

Magnetic resonance imaging

Magnetic resonance imaging (MRI) is utilized for several purposes in the diagnosis of MS (Figure 3.1). It demonstrates the presence of lesions typical of MS (Figure 3.2); by demonstrating the presence of asymptomatic lesions, it indicates whether the criteria of anatomic dissemination and development of lesions over time are satisfied. When it demonstrates lesions with imaging features atypical of MS, it points to an alternative diagnosis. Finally, in patients with known MS, MRI is used to rule out development of a superimposed disease process. Consensus guidelines for brain and spine MRI in MS have been published [1].

Typical MRI findings in MS		
Brain lesions	Signal characteristics	T2 hyperintense, T1 iso- or hypointense
	Geometry	Ovoid or patchy/irregular, discrete, or confluent
	Location	Multifocal lesions in the white and gray matter Predilection for periventricular white matter
	Locations suggestive of MS	Periventricular ovoid lesions oriented perpendicular to the ependymal surface (Dawson's fingers), corpus callosum (particularly the under-surface), subcortical U-fibers, brainstem, cerebellar peduncles, cerebellum
Gd-enhancement	Incidence	On a given scan some but not all lesions enhance
		~40–50% of patients with untreated RR MS will show Gd-enhancement on a single MRI scan
	Location	Associated with T2 hyperintensity
	Lesion enhancement pattern	Diffuse or rim
	Duration	2 out of 3 lesions enhance for 2–6 weeks, a few enhance for up to 12–16 weeks
Atrophy	Location	Parenchymal → ventricular enlargement
		Corpus callosum → thinning
		Cortical → sulcal enlargement
Cord lesions	Signal characteristics	T2 hyperintense, T1 isointense
	Geometry	Ovoid or patchy/irregular
	Location	Cervical or thoracic cord, often eccentric, extend <1 to at most several vertebral segments
	Lesion enhancement pattern	Typically diffuse or patchy, may persist for several months

Figure 3.1 Typical MRI findings in MS. Gd, gadolinium; RR, relapsing–remitting.

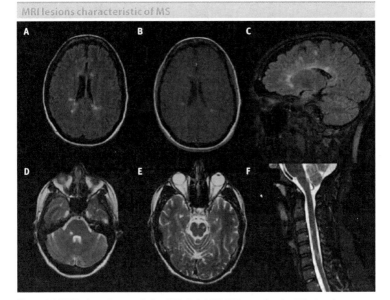

Figure 3.2 MRI lesions characteristic of MS. A, Axial FLAIR image showing T2 lesions in periventricular white matter, centrum semiovale, subcortical white matter; B, axial T1-weighted image showing rim and diffuse gadolinium-enhancing foci; C, sagittal FLAIR image showing lesions in corpus callosum; D, axial T2-weighted image showing right middle cerebellar peduncle lesion; E, axial T2-weighted image showing a left midbrain peduncle lesion; F, sagittal T2-weighted image of cervical spine showing multiple patchy lesions.

MRI also is useful to help assess the need for disease-modifying therapy by indicating both disease severity, through lesion burden and atrophy, and activity, via gadolinium (Gd)-enhancing lesions and lesion accrual. When patients have been started on therapy, MRI assists in assessing response to treatment.

Cerebrospinal fluid analysis

Cerebrospinal fluid (CSF) examination is an important ancillary test for diagnosing MS but is not mandatory in all cases. It is utilized to provide additional support for the diagnosis when clinical features and MRI are insufficient to make a definative diagnosis. CSF findings in MS are summarized in Figure 3.3. In general, the CSF picture in MS is nonspecific, but in the appropriate context, the demonstration of intrathecal antibody production (increased immunoglobulin G [IgG] index and synthesis

Typical CSF findings in MS	
Opening pressure	Normal
Glucose	Normal
Protein	Normal in 2 out of 3 patients with MS, rarely >100 mg/dL
Erythrocytes	Absent
Leukocytes	Absent in 2 out of 3 patients with MS, usually <50/mm³, rarely >100/mm³
	Predominantly mononuclear cells
Microbiologic studies	Negative
Cytology	Negative
Intrathecal antibody production	Increased total IgG, increased IgG index and synthesis rate, (+) oligoclonal bands, or increased free kappa light chains
Measures of tissue injury	Increased myelin basic protein

Figure 3.3 Typical CSF findings in MS. CSF, cerebrospinal fluid; IgG, immunoglobulin G.

rate, presence of oligoclonal bands, and increased concentration of free kappa light chains) is highly suggestive of MS. CSF examination also is used to pursue an alternative diagnosis when there are atypical clinical or MRI findings, suggesting, for example, neoplasm, infection, or cerebral vasculitis.

Evoked potentials

Evoked potentials are utilized to demonstrate subclinical involvement (slowed conduction) in CNS sensory pathways when the neurologic examination and MRI are insufficient to provide objective evidence of a multifocal disease process. Evoked potentials can be used to evaluate the afferent visual pathways (visual-evoked potentials), auditory pathways (brainstem auditory-evoked potentials), and dorsal column sensory pathways (somatosensory-evoked potentials) with median nerve (upper extremity) or posterior tibial nerve (lower extremity) stimulation. Slowing of central conduction times, particularly if asymmetric, suggests MS in the appropriate clinical setting.

Future potential of disease biomarkers in multiple sclerosis

Although increased IgG index or the presence of oligoclonal bands in the CSF are useful for supporting an MS diagnosis, and the discovery of antibodies to aquaporin-4 in patients with neuromyelitis optica (NMO) can be useful in the differential diagnosis process, there are currently no specific biomarkers to confirm a diagnosis of MS. While several candidate biomarkers in serum and CSF show promise [2,3], none so far has the validated reliability necessary for widespread clinical use.

Diagnostic criteria

There is no pathognomonic clinical, laboratory, or imaging finding or combination of findings to diagnose MS. Ultimately, making the diagnosis involves weighing the evidence supporting MS against factors suggesting a different condition. Specifically, one assembles data by evaluating the following:

- how the CNS is affected, by reviewing a patient's history, neurologic examination, MRI, and evoked potentials for evidence supporting a multifocal process (ie, dissemination in space [DIS]);
- the disease course, for example onset in a young adult of a relapsing then progressive disorder with development of lesions over time (ie, dissemination in time [DIT]);
- inflammatory features as seen through a CSF examination or MRI.
- eliminating other likely causes, for instance, by reviewing a patient's history, examinations, MRI, CSF, or blood studies.

The diagnostic logic for MS is delineated in formal diagnostic criteria developed initially for research studies. The first widely applied criteria, the Schumacher criteria proposed in 1965 [4], outlined the principles that still are used to diagnose MS: that MS is a chronic disease that first presents in young adults and evolves over time with a relapsing or progressive course. The diagnosis depended on objective evidence of development of lesions over time that was disseminated anatomically. This concept has been retained in all subsequent diagnostic criteria. The Schumacher criteria, which were proposed prior to the development of sensitive imaging techniques, depended on demonstration of objective clinical manifestations to fulfill the criterion of lesion DIT and DIS.

The Poser criteria proposed in 1983 [5] incorporated MRI and evoked potentials to demonstrate lesion dissemination and CSF examination (oligoclonal bands, or increased IgG index or synthesis rate) to provide laboratory support for the diagnosis. Clinicians often found the Poser criteria cumbersome to use in practice.

In 2001, an international panel proposed the currently used International (McDonald) Criteria [6], later revised in 2005 and again in 2010 by Polman et al [7,8]. These criteria (Figure 3.4 and 3.5) sought to retain the useful features of prior criteria but incorporated imaging more effectively into the diagnostic process, clarified definitions, simplified categories, and created a diagnostic scheme that would be useful both for research studies and clinical practice. The conceptual requirement for objective evidence of lesion DIT and DIS was maintained, but formal criteria were introduced to utilize MRI for this purpose. The 2010 revised McDonald Criteria incorporated published recommendations from the European MAGNIMS multicenter collaboration relating to the use and interpretation of imaging criteria for DIT and DIS [9,10]. These indicate that:

- DIT can be demonstrated by a new T2 or Gd-enhancing lesion on a follow-up MRI, with reference to a baseline scan, regardless of when the baseline MRI was obtained. Previous versions of the Criteria had specified that the reference scan be performed at least 30 days after the initial clinical event; this is no longer a requirement.
- DIS can be demonstrated with at least one T2 lesion in at least two out of four areas of the CNS: periventricular, juxtacortical, infratentorial, or spinal cord. These lesions need not be Gd-enhanced.

These revised DIT and DIS criteria allow for a simplified diagnostic process for MS, with equivalent or improved specificity and/or sensitivity compared with past criteria and potentially fewer required MRI examinations in many cases. In addition to the assessment of DIT and DIS, the 2010 revisions emphasized that the criteria should only be applied to patients who have experienced a typical clinically isolated syndrome (CIS) suggestive of MS, as the development and validation of the McDonald Criteria were limited to patients with such a presentation [8]. The revised guidelines also incorporated the MAGNIMS recommendations for demonstrating DIS into the diagnostic criteria for primary-progressive MS to harmonize with other 2010 updates

International criteria for the diagnosis of MS

Clinical presentation	Additional data needed for MS diagnosis
≥2 relapses; objective clinical evidence of ≥2 lesions or objective clinical evidence of 1 lesion with reasonable historical evidence of a prior relapse	None
≥2 relapses; objective clinical evidence of 1 lesion	DIS, demonstrated by MRI or a further clinical relapse
1 relapse; objective clinical evidence of ≥2 lesions	DIT, demonstrated by MRI or a further clinical relapse
1 relapse; objective clinical evidence of 1 lesion (CIS)	DIS, demonstrated by MRI or a second clinical relapse, and DIT, demonstrated by MRI or a second clinical relapse
Insidious neurologic progression suggestive of MS	1 year of disease progression plus two out of three of the following: • Evidence for DIS in the brain, demonstrated by MRI (≥1 T2 lesions) • Evidence for DIS in the spinal cord, demonstrated by MRI (≥2 T2 lesions) • Positive CSF

Figure 3.4 International criteria for the diagnosis of MS. CIS, clinically isolated syndrome; CSF, cerebrospinal fluid; DIS, dissemination in space; DIT, dissemination in time. Reproduced with permission from Polman et al [8].

International criteria for MRI findings supporting the diagnosis of MS

DIS can be demonstrated by ≥1 T2 lesion in at least two out of four of the following areas of the CNS:

- Periventricular
- Juxtacortical
- Infratentorial
- Spinal cord

DIT can be demonstrated by:

- A new T2 and/or Gd-enhancing lesion(s) on follow-up MRI, with reference to a baseline scan, irrespective of the timing of the baseline MRI
- Simultaneous presence of asymptomatic Gd-enhancing and nonenhancing lesions at any time

Figure 3.5 International criteria for MRI findings supporting the diagnosis of MS. CNS, central nervous system; DIS, dissemination in space; DIT, dissemination in time; Gd, gadolinium. Reproduced with permission from Polman et al [8].

(Figure 3.4, Figure 3.5). Furthermore, an important area of controversy related to the original McDonald Criteria was their applicability to specific populations, such as pediatric, Asian, and Latin American populations. The international panel concluded that the 2010 revised criteria were applicable to the majority of these populations once careful evaluation for other potential explanations for the clinical presentation is made. Finally, it is important to emphasize that, as with the original criteria, the 2010 revisions require testing in prospective and retrospective datasets to further assess their validity and to provide suggestions for further refinements.

Differential diagnosis

All of the diagnostic criteria include the provision that other diagnostic possibilities have been eliminated. As summarized in Figure 3.6, the potential differential diagnosis of MS is extensive [11], but not every other potential diagnosis must be pursued in every patient. Rather, the diagnostic process should be tailored to the clinical situation (Figure 3.7).

Differential diagnosis of MS

Monophasic CNS inflammatory demyelinating syndromes (ie, clinically isolated syndromes) – optic neuritis, cerebral, brainstem, partial transverse myelitis

Fulminant idiopathic CNS inflammatory syndromes – acute disseminated encephalomyelitis, Devic's neuromyelitis optica, Marburg's disease, tumefactive MS, Baló's concentric sclerosis, Schilder disease

Inflammatory/immune – systemic lupus erythematosus, Sjögren's syndrome, Behçet's syndrome, Wegener's granulomatosis, polyarteritis nodosa, isolated CNS vasculitis, Susac's syndrome, Sneddon's syndrome, sarcoid, celiac disease, stiff-person syndrome, treatment with tumor necrosis factor blockers

Infection – Lyme disease, syphilis, human immunodeficiency virus, human T cell lymphoma virus, progressive multifocal leukoencephalopathy, Whipple's disease, herpes viruses, mycoplasma, chlamydia

Vascular – small vessel ischemia, migraine, emboli, antiphospholipid antibody syndrome, cerebral autosomal dominant arteriopathy with subcortical infarcts and leukoencephalopathy, cavernous angioma of brainstem

Genetic/degenerative – mitochondrial cytopathy, hereditary spastic paraplegia, hereditary cerebellar ataxias, presenilin-I disorders, leukodystrophies, adrenomyeloneuropathy, Fabry's disease, Alexander's disease, Niemann–Pick disease, glutaryl-coenzyme A dehydrogenase deficiency, Pelizaeus–Merzbacher disease, Krabbe's disease, olivopontocerebellar atrophy, motor neuron disease, hereditary episodic ataxias

Metabolic – thyroid disease, vitamin B_{12} deficiency, nitrous oxide intoxication, copper deficiency, porphyria

Neoplastic – CNS lymphoma, intravascular lymphoma, metastasis, histiocytosis, paraneoplastic

Spine – vascular malformations, tumor, degenerative spine disease

Figure 3.6 Differential diagnosis of MS. CNS, central nervous system.

It is useful to make a preliminary determination of which of the following categories the patient belongs to before undertaking extensive testing:

1. **Clinical and imaging features "classic" for MS (ie, absence of red flags – see below).** In this setting, the diagnosis of MS is typically straightforward, and extensive testing is unnecessary. Cranial MRI and appropriate screening blood tests usually are sufficient to confirm the diagnosis.

2. **An initial episode typical of an MS relapse (ie, a CIS).** The most common CISs include optic neuritis, a cerebral syndrome, brainstem syndrome, or partial transverse myelitis. Similar to "classic" relapsing–remitting (RR) MS, extensive

Laboratory tests to assist in making the diagnosis of MS

Test	Indication	Comments
MRI	All patients	Brain MRI: to demonstrate the presence of lesions indicative of MS and the absence of findings that suggest an alternative diagnosis
		Images should include axial and sagittal fluid attenuated inversion recovery, axial T2-weighted images, and axial T1-weighted images pre/post Gd administration
	Selected patients	Spine MRI: can demonstrate the presence of lesions indicative of MS and the absence of findings suggests an alternative diagnosis
CSF examination	Selected patients	Studies should include cell count, glucose, protein, IgG index and synthesis rate, electrophoresis for oligoclonal bands to demonstrate findings indicative of MS plus additional tests tailored to the individual patient to demonstrate absence of findings suggesting an alternative diagnosis
Evoked potentials	Selected patients	Visual-, brainstem auditory-, or somatosensory-evoked potentials to confirm multifocal lesions in sensory pathways when not demonstrated by clinical features or imaging
Blood studies	All patients	Screening studies for the most common MS mimics or contributors to common symptoms: CBC, TSH, vitamin B_{12}, sedimentation rate, ANA
	Selected patients	Blood studies for specific considerations

Figure 3.7 Laboratory tests to assist in making the diagnosis of MS. ANA, antinuclear antibodies; CBC, complete blood count; CSF, cerebrospinal fluid; Gd, gadolinium; IgG, immunoglobulin G; TSH, thyroid-stimulating hormone.

testing is unnecessary in this situation; cranial MRI (plus spine MRI for cord syndromes) and screening blood studies usually suffice.

3. **MS plus an additional superimposed condition.** It is important to remain vigilant for the presence or development of an additional disease process in patients with known MS. The superimposed disorder may explain atypical manifestations or may contribute to manifestations seemingly due to MS. Thus, it is important to evaluate the principal site of neurologic disability, for example, to rule out spondylotic myelopathy in an MS patient with progressive myelopathy.

4. **A picture compatible with the diagnosis of MS but with atypical features (ie, presence of red flags).** Red flags may be demographic or clinical features (summarized in Figure 3.8), MRI findings (summarized in Figure 3.9), or CSF findings (summarized in Figure 3.10). In such patients an MS mimic needs to be considered. Additional testing tailored to the clinical situation is necessary to confirm MS and eliminate other possibilities. This scenario also includes inflammatory CNS syndromes suggesting acute disseminated encephalomyelitis, Devic's NMO, tumefactive MS, and other fulminant MS variants.

Red flags include absence of expected features, particularly in severe or long-standing disease, and presence of atypical features (ie, manifestations for which MS would be an unusual cause). They differ in their significance, that is, in how strongly they indicate that a diagnosis of MS needs to be considered and pursued. The strength of red flags varies from minor (nonspecific or weakly atypical) to major (very rare/unprecedented in MS and/or indicative of a specific other diagnosis).

Clinical red flags suggesting a diagnosis other than MS

Red flag	Examples of other diagnostic considerations
General	
Onset prior to age 20 years	Acute disseminated leukoencephalopathy, genetic disorder
Onset after age 50 years	Vascular disease
Primary progression	Structural, metabolic, degenerative, progressive multifocal leukoencephalopathy
Abrupt onset	Vascular process
Stereotypic family history	Genetic disorder, including mitochondrial, cerebral autosomal dominant arteriopathy with subcortical infarcts and leukoencephalopathy
Neurologic manifestations	
Headache, meningismus	Migraine, cerebral autosomal dominant arteriopathy with subcortical infarcts and leukoencephalopathy, chronic meningitis, sarcoid, vasculitis
Multiple cranial neuropathies, polyradiculopathy	Chronic meningitis
Peripheral neuropathy	Leukodystrophy, including adrenoleukodystrophy, vitamin B_{12} deficiency, nitrous oxide intoxication, copper deficiency
Pyramidal alone	Motor neuron disease, hereditary spastic paraparesis, syringomyelia, stiff-person
Ataxia alone	Paraneoplastic syndrome, spinocerebellar atrophy, olivopontocerebellar atrophy, celiac disease
Extrapyramidal	Olivopontocerebellar atrophy, Whipple's disease
Hearing loss	Susac's syndrome, chronic meningitis
Persistently monofocal manifestations	Structural, vascular
Systemic manifestations	
Constitutional symptoms	Cancer, sarcoid, Whipple's disease
Arthralgias, myalgias	Connective tissue disorder, Lyme disease, chronic fatigue syndrome/ fibromyalgia, Whipple's disease, Behçet's syndrome
Sicca syndrome	Sjögren's syndrome
Rash	Lyme disease, systemic lupus erythematosus, vasculitis, herpes zoster, Rocky Mountain spotted fever
Livedo reticularis	Antiphospholipid antibody syndrome
Miscarriages	Antiphospholipid antibody syndrome
Thromboembolic events	Antiphospholipid antibody syndrome, endocarditis, atrial fibrillation
Mucosal ulcers	Behçet's syndrome
Gastrointestinal symptoms	Celiac disease, vitamin B_{12} deficiency, copper deficiency, Whipple's disease
History of gastrointestinal bypass surgery	Vitamin B_{12} deficiency, copper deficiency
Retinopathy	Susac's syndrome, vasculitis, diabetes, paraneoplastic syndrome, mitochondrial disorder, sarcoid
Uveitis	Connective tissue disorder, lymphoma, sarcoid, Lyme disease
Cardiac disease	Lyme disease, emboli, endocarditis, mitochondrial

Figure 3.8 Clinical red flags suggesting a diagnosis other than MS.

MRI findings in selected mimics of MS (MRI red flags)

Disorder	MRI features
Infectious	
Lyme disease	Multifocal white and gray matter lesions
Progressive multifocal leukoencephalopathy	Confluent, gradually enlarging T2-hyperintense T1-hypointense lesions in cerebrum and posterior fossa, without Gd-enhancement or faint enhancement of leading edge
	Patchy Gd-enhancement with immune reconstitution
Human T cell lymphoma virus	Spinal cord atrophy, sparse cerebral lesions
Inflammatory	
Connective tissue disorders	Subcortical or gray matter lesions
Isolated angiitis of the nervous system	Ischemic lesions, infarcts, gray matter lesions, vascular or meningeal Gd-enhancement
Sarcoid	Mass lesions, persistent lesion Gd-enhancement, vascular or meningeal Gd-enhancement
Behçet's syndrome	Predominantly brainstem involvement
Neoplastic	
CNS lymphoma	Single or multiple lesions in gray matter, white matter, corpus callosum; lesions with mass effect, progressive enlargement, persistent Gd-enhancement; Gd-enhancement of all lesions; vascular Gd-enhancement
Metabolic, hereditary, degenerative	
Vitamin B_{12} deficiency	Diffuse abnormal T2 hyperintensity in posterior cervical cord, punctate or patchy cerebral lesions
Leukodystrophies	Diffuse abnormal T2 hyperintensity in cerebral white matter
Mitochondrial	Transient gray or white matter lesions, basal ganglia calcifications
Cerebral autosomal dominant arteriopathy with subcortical infarcts and leukoencephalopathy	Infarcts, microhemorrhages, T2 hyperintensity in temporal white matter and external capsule
Motor neuron disease	Abnormal T2 hyperintensity in corticospinal tracts
Spinocerebellar atrophy	Cerebellar, brainstem, cord atrophy with normal T2 signal
Spine disease	
Dural arteriovenous malformation	Patchy T2 hyperintensity and/or swelling in cord, persistent faint Gd-enhancement, draining veins
Degenerative spine disease	Spondylosis and/or herniated disc with cord decompression and associated myelomalacia

Figure 3.9 MRI findings in selected mimics of MS (MRI red flags). CNS, central nervous system; Gd, gadolinium.

Red flag	Examples of other diagnostic considerations
Increased opening pressure	Chronic meningitis
Decreased glucose	Chronic meningitis
Protein >100 mg/dL	Chronic meningitis, sarcoid, vasculitis, cord compression
White blood count >100/mm³	Chronic meningitis, sarcoid, vasculitis
White blood cell differential with neutrophils	Acute infection
White blood cell differential with eosinophils	Vasculitis, parasitic infection
Cytology with cellular atypia	Metastases, CNS lymphoma, glial neoplasm
Lack of intrathecal antibody production	Nonimmune condition

CSF red flags suggesting a diagnosis other than MS

Figure 3.10 CSF red flags suggesting a diagnosis other than MS. CNS, central nervous system.

References

1 Simon JH, Li D, Traboulsee A, et al. Standardized MR imaging protocol for multiple sclerosis: Consortium of MS Centers consensus guidelines. *AJNR Am J Neuroradiol.* 2006;27:455-461.

2 Awad A, Hemmer B, Hartung HP, et al. Analyses of cerebrospinal fluid in the diagnosis and monitoring of multiple sclerosis. *J Neuroimmunol.* 2010;219:1-7.

3 Quintana FJ, Farez MF, Viglietta V, et al. Antigen microarrays identify unique serum autoantibody signatures in clinical and pathologic subtypes of multiple sclerosis. *Proc Natl Acad Sci USA.* 2008;105:18889-18894.

4 Schumacher GA, Beebe GW, Kibler RF, et al. Problems of experimental trials of therapy in multiple sclerosis: Report by the panel on the evaluation of experimental trials of therapy in multiple sclerosis. *Ann N Y Acad Sci.* 1965;122:552-568.

5 Poser C, Paty D, Scheinberg L, et al. New diagnostic criteria for multiple sclerosis: guidelines for research protocols. *Ann Neurol.* 1983;13:227-231.

6 McDonald WI, Compston DA, Edan G, et al. Recommended diagnostic criteria for multiple sclerosis: guidelines from the International Panel on the Diagnosis of Multiple Sclerosis. *Ann Neurol.* 2001;50:121-127.

7 Polman CH, Reingold SC, Edan G, et al. Diagnostic criteria for multiple sclerosis: 2005 revisions to the "McDonald Criteria". *Ann Neurol.* 2005;58:840-846.

8 Polman CH, Reingold SC, Banwell B, et al. Diagnostic criteria for multiple sclerosis: 2010 revisions to the McDonald Criteria. *Ann Neurol.* 2011;69:292-302.

9 Swanton JK, Rovira A, Tintoré M, et al. MRI criteria for multiple sclerosis in patients presenting with clinically isolated syndromes: a multicentre retrospective study. *Lancet Neurol.* 2007;6:677-686.

10 Swanton JK, Fernando K, Dalton CM, et al. Modification of MRI criteria for multiple sclerosis in patients with clinically isolated syndromes. *J Neurol Neurosurg Psychiatry.* 2006;77:830-833.

11 Miller DH, Weinshenker BG, Filippi M, et al. Differential diagnosis of suspected multiple sclerosis: a consensus approach. *Mult Scler.* 2008;14:1157-1174.

Treatment of acute relapses of multiple sclerosis

The evaluation and treatment of acute multiple sclerosis (MS) relapses has several aspects:

- Evaluation of the patient to determine whether the change in neurologic status represents a bona fide relapse and whether an intercurrent medical condition (eg, infection) may have triggered the relapse. MS relapses must be distinguished from transient day-to-day fluctuations in neurologic symptoms common in patients with MS, pseudo-relapses (worsening of pre-existing neurologic manifestations in association with a febrile illness or metabolic derangement), or progression (gradual worsening over months).
- Treatment of underlying infection or metabolic derangement if one is identified.
- Symptomatic therapy (eg, for vertigo from a brainstem relapse).
- A short course of corticosteroids to accelerate recovery and, in theory, improve degree of recovery.
- Rehabilitation to develop compensatory strategies (eg, for gait impairment and to promote functional recovery).
- Reconsideration of long-term disease therapy: the occurrence of a relapse may indicate the need to initiate or alter disease-modifying therapy.
- Magnetic resonance imaging (MRI) on a case-by-case basis; typically it is not necessary to perform MRI to diagnose an acute

J. A. Cohen and A. Rae-Grant, *Handbook of Multiple Sclerosis*,
DOI: 10.1007/978-1-907673-50-4_4, © Springer Healthcare 2012

relapse. MRI is sometimes obtained in the setting of a suspected acute relapse to rule out an alternative explanation for the change in neurologic status. It also may be useful to assess the level of disease activity to guide the decision to initiate or alter disease therapy.

Short courses of high-dose corticosteroids are routinely used to treat acute MS relapses. The principal purpose of corticosteroid therapy is to accelerate recovery [1]. Theoretical goals include limiting damage, improving the degree of recovery, and delaying the next relapse. Some but not all studies support these additional goals. Typically, relapses that cause significant impairment and interfere with daily function and/or are failing to improve spontaneously are treated, unless there is a strong contraindication to corticosteroids. Mild relapses that are already improving may not require treatment. In general, treatment should be started as soon as a relapse is confirmed, although a delay of several days usually is not problematic. An exception is Devic's neuromyelitis optica (NMO), which often evolves rapidly, is fulminant, and tends to recover incompletely. Therefore, therapy for relapses in NMO should be initiated as soon as a relapse is suspected.

The typical corticosteroid regimen employed at the Mellen Center at the Cleveland Clinic is methylprednisolone 1000 mg administered intravenously as a single daily dose on 3 consecutive days in an outpatient setting, with a subsequent 12-day tapering dose of oral prednisone: 60 mg/day for 4 days, 40 mg/day for 4 days, and 20 mg/day for 4 days. Potential modifications of the standard regimen in selected situations are summarized in Figure 4.1. Relapses that fail to respond to a standard course of intravenous methlyprednisolone can be treated by repeating intravenous methlyprednisolone (extending the second course to 5–7 days) or plasma exchange [2].

Short courses of high-dose corticosteroids generally are safe and well tolerated. However, potential adverse effects are myriad [3]. The most common adverse effects associated with short courses of corticosteroids (both intravenous and oral) include metallic taste, insomnia, dysphoria, anxiety, increased appetite, edema, headache, myalgia, easy bruising, acne, gastrointestinal distress/heartburn, flushing, and palpitations.

Potential modifications of the standard corticosteroid regimen used to treat MS relapses

Reduced methylprednisolone dose – Some patients, including those with small body mass, tolerate a lower dose better (eg, 500 mg/dose)

Dosing interval – Some patients tolerate divided doses of methlyprednisolone better (eg, 250 mg every 6 hours)

Treatment duration – For more severe relapses or relapses that are not improving, the duration of intravenous methlyprednisolone sometimes is extended to 5–7 days

Oral prednisone taper – Typically, the dose is tapered to lessen rebound symptoms, except in patients with known poor tolerability from side effects or a complicating condition (eg, diabetes, hypertension, or osteoporosis). The taper is usually over 12 days but may be more rapid to lessen adverse effects or more prolonged in patients with a known tendency to experience rebound symptoms with the standard taper

Corticosteroids – Limited experience suggests other corticosteroids (eg, dexamethasone at comparable doses) are equally efficacious

Treatment setting – Relapses are routinely treated in an outpatient setting, in an infusion center or at home via homecare. A patient's first course of intravenous methylprednisolone typically is administered under observation in a medical setting until tolerability is confirmed. Patients are hospitalized if felt to be unsafe at home due to neurologic manifestations (eg, inability to walk), require symptomatic therapy (eg, intravenous fluids for vertigo with nausea and dehydration), or to manage steroid complications (eg, hyperglycemia or severe mood disorder/psychosis)

Figure 4.1 Potential modifications of the standard corticosteroid regimen used to treat MS relapses.

Uncommon but important adverse effects associated with short courses of corticosteroids include anaphylaxis, osteonecrosis/aseptic necrosis of joints, psychosis, euphoria, depression, and exacerbation of pre-existing peptic ulcer disease, diabetes mellitus, hypertension, and affective disorders. Chronic corticosteroids increase the risk of bone mineral density loss, cataracts, fatty liver, Cushingoid habitus, infection diathesis, and impaired healing. Several studies have shown that intermittent, short courses of corticosteroids to treat MS are not associated with a significantly increased risk of these conditions [4]. Approaches to address corticosteroid-related side effects are listed in Figure 4.2.

Several studies and clinical experience suggest that low-dose oral prednisone (approximately 1 mg/kg/day) is not as effective as intravenous methylprednisolone at the usual dose of 1000 mg/day to treat acute MS relapses [5]. Therefore, relapses typically are not treated with low-dose oral prednisone alone. Substantial evidence supports the substitution of comparable doses of oral corticosteroids for high-dose intravenous

Approaches to treat corticosteroid-related side effects

Diet – Patients are advised a diet with no concentrated sweets (to lessen risk of hyperglycemia), no added salt (to decrease fluid retention), and foods rich in potassium (to prevent hypokalemia)

Gastrointestinal prophylaxis – Typically, famotidine 20 mg once or twice daily is prescribed to lessen risk of gastritis, although there are limited data confirming benefit

Insomnia – Patients frequently experience insomnia during corticosteroid treatment and are typically managed by providing a short-acting hypnotic to be taken at bedtime

Hyperglycemia – Blood sugar should be monitored in patients with known diabetes mellitus or past history of corticosteroid-associated hyperglycemia. It usually is advisable to involve the patient's primary care provider

Hypertension – Blood pressure should be monitored, particularly in patients with known essential or corticosteroid-associated hypertension. It usually is advisable to involve the patient's primary care provider

Mood disorder – Mood should be monitored, particularly in patients with known affective disorder

Patient education – Informing patients about potential corticosteroid side effects is an important aspect of relapse management

Figure 4.2 Approaches to treat corticosteroid-related side effects.

methlyprednisolone. Arguments in favor include feasibility (comparable doses can be administered orally), greater convenience, reduced cost [6], comparable bioavailability [7], good tolerability [8], and reported equivalence in other disorders, such as asthma [9] and rheumatoid arthritis [10]. Comparable high doses of oral and intravenous steroids have been reported to have similar benefit in treating MS relapses in several small studies [11–15]. An adequately sized study to confirm equivalence has not been done. At the Mellen Center, typically acute MS relapses are treated with intravenous methlyprednisolone. However, high-dose oral corticosteroids are used in certain situations, such as poor venous access, needle phobia, or lack of insurance coverage for intravenous infusion. Oral options include methlyprednisolone (500–1000 mg/day) or prednisone (1250 mg/day).

References

1   Miller D, Weinstock-Guttman B, Bethoux F, et al. A meta-analysis of methylprednisolone in recovery from multiple sclerosis exacerbations. *Mult Scler.* 2000;6:267-273.
2   Weinshenker BG, O'Brien P, Petterson TM, et al. A randomized trial of plasma exchange in acute central nervous system inflammatory demyelinating disease. *Ann Neurol.*1999;46:878-886.

3   Fox RJ, Kinkel RP. High-dose methylprednisolone in the treatment of multiple sclerosis. In: Cohen JA, Rudick RA, eds. *Multiple Sclerosis Therapeutics, 3rd edition*. London, UK: Informa Healthcare; 2007:515-533.

4   Cohen JA, Imrey PB, Calabresi PA, et al. Results of the Avonex Combination Trial (ACT) in relapsing–remitting MS. *Neurology*. 2009;72:535-541.

5   Beck RW, Cleary PA, Anderson MM, et al. A randomized, controlled trial of corticosteroids in the treatment of acute optic neuritis. *N Engl J Med*. 1992;326:581-588.

6   Robson LS, Bain C, Beck S, et al. Cost analysis of methylprednisolone treatment of multiple sclerosis patients. *Can J Neurol Sci*. 1998;25:222-229.

7   Morrow SA, Stoian CA, Dmitrovic J, et al. The bioavailability of IV methylprednisolone and oral prednisone in multiple sclerosis. *Neurology*. 2004;63:1079-1080.

8   Metz LM, Sabuda D, Hilsden RJ, et al. Gastric tolerance of high-dose pulse oral prednisone n multiple sclerosis. *Neurology*. 1999;53:2093-2096.

9   Ratto D, Alfaro C, Sipsey J, et al. Are intravenous corticosteroids required in status asthmaticus? *JAMA*. 1988;260:527-529.

10 Smith MD, Ahern MJ, Roberts-Thomson PJ. Pulse steroid therapy in rheumatoid arthritis: can equivalent doses of oral prednisolone give similar clinical results to intravenous methylprednisolone? *Ann Rheum Dis*. 1988;47:28-33.

11 Alam SM, Kyriakides T, Lawden M, et al. Methylprednisolone in multiple sclerosis: a comparison of oral with intravenous therapy at equivalent high dose. *J Neurol Neurosurg Psychiatry*. 1993;56:1219-1220.

12 Barnes D, Hughes RAC, Morris RW, et al. Randomised trial of oral and intravenous methylprednisolone in acute relapses of multiple sclerosis. *Lancet*. 1997;349:902-906.

13 Sellebjerg F, Frederiksen JL, Nielsen PM, et al. Double-blind, randomized, placebo-controlled study of oral, high-dose methylprednisolone in attacks of MS. *Neurology*. 1998;51:529-534.

14 Sellebjerg F, Nielsen SH, Fredericksen JL, et al. A randomized, controlled trial of oral high-dose methylprednisolone in acute optic neuritis. *Neurology*. 1999;52:1479-1484.

15 Martinelli V, Rocca MA, Annovazzi P, et al. A short-term randomized MRI study of high-dose oral vs intravenous methylprednisolone in MS. *Neurology*. 2009;73:1842-1848.

Chapter 5

Disease-modifying therapy

Disease-modifying agents

Since 1993 eight disease-modifying agents have been approved by regulatory agencies to treat relapsing–remitting multiple sclerosis (RR MS) (see Figure 5.1). In addition, a sizable number of agents are used off label alone or in combination.

Glatiramer acetate

Glatiramer acetate is a complex mixture of random synthetic polypeptides that probably functions as an altered peptide ligand for the major histocompatibility complex (MHC) class II molecules and, when presented to T cells, inhibits activation and induces regulatory cells [1]. Glatiramer acetate may also stimulate neuroprotective and/or repair mechanisms. Two Phase III studies demonstrated that glatiramer acetate 20 mg administered by daily subcutaneous injection reduced relapses in RR MS [2,3], with a reduction of approximately 30% in the second study. A separate randomized controlled trial confirmed the beneficial effect on relapses and demonstrated a benefit in terms of magnetic resonance imaging (MRI) measures, including gadolinium (Gd)-enhancing lesions, new T2 lesions, and the proportion of lesions evolving into T1-hypointense "black holes" [4,5]. Glatiramer acetate is therefore currently approved in the USA, EU, and many other countries for RR MS, at the recommended daily dose of 20 mg subcutaneously. The ongoing GALA study is assessing a lower frequency dosing regimen of glatiramer

J. A. Cohen and A. Rae-Grant, *Handbook of Multiple Sclerosis*,
DOI: 10.1007/978-1-907673-50-4_5, © Springer Healthcare 2012

Approved disease-modifying medications for relapsing MS

Agent	Dose	Approved MS indications	Principal adverse effects	Laboratory monitoring	Pregnancy category*
Glatiramer acetate (Copaxone®)	20 mg SC daily	USA: CIS, RR MS CN: CIS, RR MS EU: CIS, RR MS	Injection site reaction, immediate post-injection reactions (flushing, dyspnea, palpitations, diaphoresis, anxiety)	None	B
Interferon β-1a (Avonex®)	30 μg IM weekly	USA: CIS, relapsing forms of MS CN: CIS, RR MS, SP MS with relapses EU: CIS, relapsing forms of MS	Flu-like symptoms, depression, headache, leukopenia, liver abnormality, thyroid dysfunction	CBC, ALT, AST prior to therapy; months 1, 3, 6; then every 6–12 months NAb with active disease	C
Interferon β-1a (Rebif®)	22 or 44 μg SC three times per week	USA: relapsing forms of MS CN: relapsing forms of MS EU: MS with ≥2 relapses in 2 years	Flu-like symptoms, injection site reaction, depression, headache, leukopenia, liver abnormality, thyroid dysfunction	CBC, ALT, AST prior to therapy; months 1, 3, 6; then every 6–12 months NAb after 1–2 years of therapy, particularly with active disease	C
Interferon β-1b (Betaseron®)	8 MIU SC every other day	USA: CIS, relapsing forms of MS CN: CIS, RR MS, SP MS EU: CIS, RR MS, SP MS	Flu-like symptoms, injection site reaction, depression, headache, leukopenia, liver abnormality, thyroid dysfunction	CBC, ALT, AST prior to therapy; months 1, 3, 6; then every 6–12 months NAb after 1–2 years of therapy, particularly with active disease	C
Interferon β-1b (Extavia®)	8 MIU SC every other day	USA: CIS, relapsing forms of MS CN: n/a EU: CIS, RR MS, SP MS	Flu-like symptoms, injection site reaction, depression, headache, leukopenia, liver abnormality, thyroid dysfunction	CBC, ALT, AST prior to therapy; months 1, 3, 6; then every 6–12 months NAb after 1–2 years of therapy, particularly with active disease	C

Figure 5.1 Approved disease-modifying medications for relapsing MS (continues opposite).

Agent	Dose	Approved MS indications	Principal adverse effects	Laboratory monitoring	Pregnancy category*
Mitoxantrone (Novantrone®)	12 mg/m² IV every 3 months (maximum 140 mg/m²)	USA: SP MS, worsening RR MS CN: n/a EU: varies country to country but, in general, active RR or SP MS	Blue sclera and urine, nausea, alopecia, amenorrhea, infertility, leukopenia, thrombocytopenia, cardiotoxicity, leukemia	CBC and LVEF prior to every dose	D
Natalizumab (Tysabri®)	300 mg IV monthly	USA: relapsing forms of MS CN: RR MS EU: highly active RR MS	Headache, allergic reaction, liver abnormality, PML	MRI prior to therapy then every 6–12 months NAb after 6–12 months of therapy, particularly with active disease	C
Fingolimod (Gilenya®)	0.5 mg/day, oral	USA: RR MS CN: RR MS EU: RR MS	Lymphopenia, decreased heart rate, macular edema, hepatotoxicity, infection	Before first dose electrocardiogram, ophthalmology appointment and ocular coherence tomography, CBC, and CMP. If no history of chicken pox, Varicella zoster titers Ocular coherence tomography and eye exam at 4 months Recommend CBC and CMP every 3 months but no guidelines	C

Figure 5.1 Approved disease-modifying medications for relapsing MS (continued).
*For all agents, a pregnancy test is recommended in women of child-bearing potential prior to therapy and for suspected pregnancy on therapy. ALT, alanine transaminase; AST, aspartate transaminase; CBC, complete blood count; CIS, clinically isolated syndrome; CMP, comprehensive metabolic panel; CN, Canada; EU, European Union; IM, intramuscular; IV, intravenous; LVEF, left ventricular ejection fraction; NAb, neutralizing antibody; PML, progressive multifocal leukoencephalopathy; RR, relapsing–remitting; SC, subcutaneous; SP, secondary progressive; USA, United States of America.

acetate (40 mg administered three times a week) compared with placebo in patients with RR MS. In addition to its efficacy in RR MS, glatiramer acetate was shown to delay the onset of clinically definite MS in patients with clinically isolated syndrome (CIS) in a randomized, multinational Phase III study and this agent is therefore also approved as a treatment in this setting [6]. Glatiramer acetate is not approved for the treatment of progressive forms of MS.

Glatiramer acetate is generally well-tolerated. The most common side effects are injection-site erythema, induration, pruritus, or tenderness. Lipoatrophy (loss of subcutaneous fat with scarring) sometimes occurs with prolonged treatment. Its significance is primarily cosmetic, but it is typically irreversible. Glatiramer acetate rarely causes a post-injection systemic reaction comprising various combinations of flushing, diaphoresis, chest tightness, dyspnea, palpitations, and anxiety, beginning within minutes of injection and resolving spontaneously in 1–30 minutes. This reaction typically occurs once or at most a few times in a given patient and does not recur even with continued dosing. Its etiology remains uncertain, but it does not appear to represent a hypersensitivity reaction, bronchospasm, or cardiac compromise. Patients should be advised of this potential reaction. In contrast to interferon-beta (IFN-β), glatiramer acetate is not associated with constitutional side effects, depression, liver enzyme abnormalities, low blood counts, worsening headaches and spasticity, or neutralizing antibodies (NAbs).

Interferon-beta

Four IFN-β preparations have regulatory approval to treat MS: two preparations of subcutaneous IFN-β-1b, one of intramuscular IFN-β-1a, and one of subcutaneous IFN-β-1a. IFN-β modulates T and B cell function, decreases expression of matrix metalloproteinases, reverses blood–brain barrier disruption, and alters expression of a number of cytokines [1]. A series of Phase III studies in RR MS support the benefit of IFN-β in reducing relapses (by approximately 30%), disability progression, and MRI lesion activity and accrual [7–15].

Although side effects frequently occur with administration of IFN-β preparations, these agents generally are well tolerated. The most common side effects include flu-like constitutional symptoms (fever, chills, malaise, myalgias), sometimes with concomitant worsening of pre-existing neurologic symptoms. These symptoms usually last from several to 24 hours following injection, are worse with the initiation of therapy, and attenuate over time. Other side effects include injection site reactions with subcutaneous forms, rare skin necrosis, depression, leukopenia, liver abnormalities, and thyroid disorders. Patients with pre-existing headache syndromes or spasticity may experience worsening with IFN-β therapy.

Natalizumab

Natalizumab is a humanized monoclonal antibody that binds α_4 integrin and blocks interaction of $\alpha_4\beta_1$ integrin on leukocytes with vascular cell adhesion molecule and fibronectin CS1 sites on vascular endothelial cells [16]. As a result, migration of leukocytes from the blood into the central nervous system (CNS) is inhibited. A Phase III trial in RR MS showed that monthly intravenous infusions of 300 mg natalizumab reduced relapse rates by 68% over 2 years, disability progression by 42%, and MRI Gd-enhancing lesion number by 92% [17,18]. A second Phase III study supported these results, showing that natalizumab combined with intramuscular IFN-β-1a was more effective than IFN-β-1a plus placebo infusions [19].

Natalizumab generally is well tolerated. In the pivotal trials, side effects that were significantly associated with natalizumab included fatigue, anxiety, pharyngitis, sinus congestion, peripheral edema, and mild infusion-related symptoms, such as headache, flushing, erythema, nausea, fatigue, and dizziness. Allergic hypersensitivity reactions, including urticaria, pruritus, anaphylaxis, and anaphylactoid syndromes, occurred in 4% of natalizumab-treated patients and were serious in 1%. Approximately 6% of patients develop persistent anti-natalizumab NAbs [20]. In addition to abrogating the efficacy of natalizumab, the presence of NAbs increases the risk for hypersensitivity reactions. Rare hepatotoxicity has been reported, usually at the initiation of therapy.

The principal safety concern with natalizumab is increased risk for progressive multifocal leukoencephalopathy (PML), a serious and often fatal opportunistic infection of oligodendrocytes caused by reactivation of latent JC polyomavirus. In 2005, shortly after being licensed for use, natalizumab was withdrawn from the market when three fatal cases of PML were reported in patients receiving natalizumab. A subsequent safety evaluation of the drug estimated the risk of PML to be 1 in 1000 over an 18-month treatment period [21], which so far has been supported by the post-marketing experience. Following this report, natalizumab was reapproved as monotherapy for active MS in July 2006. Patients receiving natalizumab require close monitoring for PML. Formal guidelines are provided in the USA by the Tysabri Outreach: Unified Commitment to Health (TOUCH) risk management program, which requires direct questioning of the patient at each infusion for symptoms suggestive of PML. At the Mellen Center, MRI is performed prior to treatment and every 6 months. Manifestations that suggest PML include subacutely worsening visual, motor, or cognitive changes and/or gradually enlarging T2 hyperintensities with minimal or no Gd-enhancement. If PML is suspected, natalizumab treatment should be suspended, MRI should be obtained, and cerebrospinal fluid (CSF) examination performed, including polymerase chain reaction for JC virus. Repeat CSF examination may be required if there is a high level of suspicion but initial testing is negative. Brain biopsy is necessary in some patients; for example, where the diagnosis cannot be confirmed by MRI and CSF testing. At present, immune reconstitution is the main therapy for PML. Pharmacokinetic studies have shown that plasma exchange accelerates removal of natalizumab from the blood [22]. The recommended protocol is five exchanges every other day.

PML is mainly seen in conditions associated with impaired cellular immunity, including, for instance, acquired immune deficiency syndrome, cancer, and immunosuppressant therapy. The risk is very low in the first year and increases in years 2 and 3. It remains uncertain whether the risk continues to increase subsequently. Identification of MS patients that have been exposed to JC virus may also identify those at increased risk for developing PML. Data from the ongoing STRATIFY-1 study in RR MS patients who are being treated or considering treatment with natalizumab showed that a novel two-step antibody assay was able to detect anti-JC virus antibodies in serum, suggesting the potential utility of this assay as a PML risk stratification tool when used with other clinical data from the patient [23]. In January 2012, the US label for natalizumab was updated with the information that a positive test for anti-JC virus antibodies represented a risk factor for developing PML in patients treated with natalizumab for MS. Prior immunosuppressive therapy also appears to be an important PML risk factor.

Natalizumab is generally considered for patients who have relapsing MS and continued disease activity despite use of one or more of the standard disease therapies or who cannot tolerate the standard agents [24]. It also can be considered for patients with disease characteristics that suggest high risk of disability and for whom a more potent though potentially more risky agent is felt to be appropriate.

Mitoxantrone

Mitoxantrone is an anthracenedione chemotherapeutic agent that intercalates into and cross-links DNA, interfering with DNA repair and RNA synthesis. The benefit in MS derives from its potent effects on cellular and humoral immunity. Mitoxantrone was approved by the US Food and Drug Administration (FDA) in 2000 for the treatment of secondary progressive (SP) MS and worsening RR MS. In clinical trials, mitoxantrone produced prominent beneficial effects on the number of relapses and on progression of disability in patients with worsening MS [25–28]. Surprisingly, the benefit in terms of MRI outcomes was somewhat less prominent [29]. The 12-mg/m^2 dose showed greater efficacy than 5 mg/m^2 on some but not all clinical and MRI outcomes.

The approved dose of mitoxantrone is 12 mg/m^2 administered by intravenous infusion every 3 months up to a maximum dose of 140 mg/m^2. Monthly infusions of mitoxantrone for 3–6 months as induction therapy followed by a standard agent also have been utilized.

Mitoxantrone is generally well tolerated [30]. The most common side effects include blue discoloration of sclera and urine, nausea, alopecia, bone marrow suppression, amenorrhea, and infertility. Nausea, alopecia, and bone marrow suppression generally are mild compared to other chemotherapeutic agents. Prolonged amenorrhea occurs in 7% of younger women, and permanent amenorrhea occurs in up to 14% of women over the age of 35 years.

The principal dose-limiting toxicity is vacuolar cardiomyopathy [31,32], for which the risk is proportional to total lifetime cumulative dose. Therefore, it is recommended that the total cumulative dose should not exceed 140 mg/m^2. However, there have been reports of decreased cardiac function with doses less than 100 mg/m^2 and in several patients after only a few doses [32–34]. Current guidelines recommend evaluation of left ventricular ejection fraction by radionuclide ventriculography (multiple-gated acquisition scan) or echocardiography, prior to therapy initiation and every subsequent dose. Mitoxantrone should not be administered to any patient with a baseline ejection fraction less than 50% or with a 10% decrease in ejection fraction between visits, except with consultation of a cardiologist. The other emerging concern is treatment-related acute myelocytic or promyelocytic leukemia [35,36]. Because both delayed cardiotoxic effects and leukemia occur, monitoring must continue after cessation of therapy. In general, because of potential toxicity, mitoxantrone is appropriate for patients who are considered to be at risk for disability and who experience continued relapses and MRI activity or intolerable side effects on a standard agent.

Fingolimod

Fingolimod was the first oral drug to receive North American and European regulatory approval to reduce relapses in patients with RR MS. This agent is licensed for first-line therapy in the USA, but only for highly active MS and second-line therapy in Europe. Fingolimod is a sphingosine-1-phosphate receptor 1 (S1P1) modulator and has strong immunoregulatory features [37]. Through its modulatory effects on S1P1 receptors, fingolimod inhibits the migration of T cells from lymphoid tissue into the peripheral circulation and target organs, including the CNS, thus attenuating inflammation. Two Phase III studies (FREEDOMS, a placebo-controlled 24-month trial, and TRANSFORMS, a 12-month trial with comparator IFN-β-1a) demonstrated that orally administered fingolimod (0.5 mg/day and 1.25 mg/day) was effective at reducing relapses in patients with RR MS [38,39]. Furthermore, MRI-related endpoints were improved with fingolimod in both studies. Although fingolimod is generally well tolerated, specific safety issues have been identified (eg, the possible risk of herpes virus dissemination, macular edema, long-term consequences of elevated blood pressure) and these potential risks should be carefully considered. In addition, recent deaths soon after initial dosing are being reviewed by regulatory agencies and may affect safety measures related to this medication. More long-term data are needed to further assess the safety profile of fingolimod. Currently, there are no established clinical guidelines for the use of fingolimod in patients with MS but, with the relative paucity of long-term safety investigations, it has been suggested that this agent should be reserved as a second-line drug [37].

Neutralizing antibodies

NAbs are antibodies that are induced by treatment with a biologic therapy (including IFN-β and monoclonal antibodies, such as natalizumab) and interfere with its biologic actions. As a result, in MS, NAbs block the pharmacodynamic, MRI, and clinical effects of the agent. Although the significance of IFN-β NAbs remains somewhat contentious, we agree, in general, with the conclusions and recommendations of the European Federation of Neurological Societies [40]:

- The frequency of NAbs differs among IFN-β preparations. After 6–18 months of therapy the incidence is 5% with intramuscular IFN-β-1a, 25% with subcutaneous IFN-β-1a, and 35% with IFN-β-1b.
- NAbs elicited by one IFN-β preparation cross-react with other IFN-βs.
- NAb testing should be routinely performed after 12 and 24 months of IFN-β therapy and can be discontinued after that in patients who remain NAb-negative. Measurement should be repeated 3–6 months later in NAb-positive patients.
- IFN-β therapy should be discontinued in patients with persistent high-titer NAbs, regardless of apparent clinical stability.

NAbs develop in approximately 6% of natalizumab-treated patients, almost always between 6 and 9 months of treatment [20]. Anti-natalizumab NAbs abrogate the clinical and MRI effects of natalizumab, and increase the risk of hypersensitivity reactions. NAbs should be checked in patients on natalizumab after 6–12 months of therapy, particularly if there is ongoing clinical or MRI activity. Therapy should be changed in patients with persistent high-titer NAbs.

Initiating, monitoring, and changing therapy in relapsing–remitting multiple sclerosis

Initiating therapy

There is general consensus that disease therapy should be commenced in most patients with RR MS once the diagnosis has been confirmed and in selected patients with CIS who, because of the presence of multiple lesions on MRI, are considered to be at high risk of developing MS [41]. The short-term goals of disease therapy in CIS and RR MS are to reduce MRI lesion activity, the frequency and severity of relapses, and worsening impairment from relapses. There are robust data supporting the efficacy of disease therapies for these goals. The long-term goal is to delay or prevent evolution to SP MS and development of permanent disability. Although it is likely that the demonstrated short-term actions of disease therapies will translate into clinically meaningful long-term benefit, this assumption is as yet unproven.

There are no definitive guidelines to assist clinicians in selecting the agent with which to initiate therapy. Some [9,13,15,42–45], although not all [46], prospective studies support a dose effect for IFN-β. Overall, the data suggest that frequency of administration is more important than injected dose. However, the potential efficacy advantage of the higher dose/more frequently administered IFN-β preparations has several caveats. First, the reported differences in efficacy were small. Second, greater efficacy may be accompanied by increased side effects and laboratory abnormalities, and less convenience. Third, and probably most important, IFN-β-1b and subcutaneous IFN-β-1a have a substantially greater tendency than intramuscular IFN-β-1a to elicit NAbs [40,47], which abrogate their biologic activity and clinical efficacy [40]. Studies comparing IFN-β with glatiramer acetate failed to demonstrate a difference in clinical efficacy [48,49]. In general, glatiramer acetate has fewer side effects than IFN-β. However, it has the most frequent injection schedule, and its onset of action, as reflected by MRI lesion activity

[4], may be more gradual. In most circumstances, any IFN-β preparation or glatiramer acetate are reasonable options for initial therapy. A subcutaneous agent should be selected for patients on anticoagulation. In patients with a severe pre-existing headache syndrome, depression, spasticity, or with substantial concern about the possibility of side effects, glatiramer acetate is preferred.

Monitoring side effects and maintaining compliance

Once therapy has been initiated, it is important to take steps to maintain compliance (Figure 5.2), and patients must be monitored for toxicity. The principal anticipated side effects and laboratory abnormalities of the approved medications and the recommended safety monitoring have been summarized in Figure 5.1.

Monitoring efficacy

In addition, patients must be monitored for ongoing disease activity [50]. There are no validated criteria for judging what is unacceptable ongoing disease activity. Factors to consider include: relapse frequency, severity, and degree of recovery; extent of MRI lesion activity and persistence

Strategies to improve compliance with therapy

Maintain a therapeutic partnership between the patient, family, and care team to decide:
- Whether to initiate treatment
- Which agent to start
- When to switch therapy
- When to discontinue therapy

Effectively educate the patient and family concerning:
- Realistic goals for therapy
- Medication administration
- Side effects

Utilize a combination of approaches to educate patients and family, including face-to-face instruction, printed material, peer groups, and pharmaceutical support programs

Anticipate, monitor for, and expeditiously address side effects

Anticipate and address financial issues

Actively monitor compliance

Maintain regular facilitated communication between the patient, family, and care team to answer questions and address concerns

Figure 5.2 Strategies to improve compliance with therapy.

over multiple scans; and pre-existing impairment and/or MRI lesion burden. Based on the results of Phase III studies, approximately two out of three patients on glatiramer acetate or IFN-β will have a relapse or MRI lesion activity within 2 or 3 years of starting therapy. Since these agents do not have an immediate onset of action, it usually is appropriate to continue therapy for 6–12 months before determining whether or not they are being effective. Typically, patients will exhibit both clinical and MRI activity. However, MRI lesions may not have clinical manifestations, so ongoing MRI lesion activity in the absence of clinical relapses still requires attention, particularly with IFN-β, which should potently suppress Gd-enhancement. Conversely, in patients who appear to have very frequent relapses but stable MRI findings, an alternative explanation should be considered, for instance, pseudo-relapses, progression, or a non-MS cause for the symptoms.

The monitoring protocol must be tailored to the individual patient, in large part based on the perceived risk of future disability. Clinical assessments should be performed at the time of initiation of disease therapy to serve as a baseline for that agent, and then every 3–6 months. After several years of stability, assessments can be reduced to one to two per year with additional visits if potential issues arise. Clinical assessments should include patient self-reported status, enumeration of relapses, neurologic examination, and quantitative measures, such as the Timed 25-Foot Walk (T25FW) and 9-hole peg test. MRI should be obtained at the time of initiation of or major changes in therapy and then every 1 or 2 years. After several years of stability on a given agent, scan frequency can be decreased. If possible, scans should be obtained with consistent acquisition parameters, at the same facility, and on the same scanner, to facilitate comparison over time.

Changing therapy

There are several options for patients who experience continued disease activity after initiating therapy with a standard agent [50]. The choice depends on the baseline disease severity, extent of ongoing activity, expected tolerance of side effects, and patient preference. One option is to change to another standard agent; typically, this is the appropriate option for patients considered to be at modest risk. In general, switching class (ie, from an IFN-β to glatiramer acetate or vice versa) is more useful than switching within a class (ie, from one IFN-β to another), although some patients with continued activity on intramuscular IFN-β-1a may respond to a higher dose or higher frequency IFN-β. Importantly, patients with NAbs generated against one IFN-β are unlikely to respond to another IFN-β, so such patients should be switched to glatiramer acetate.

The second option is to escalate therapy. Currently, natalizumab is the most common therapy used in this setting. The potentially greater efficacy must be weighed against the risk for a potentially fatal adverse effect, which is PML. Fingolimod also is often used in this setting. Other potent therapy options include mitoxantrone, cyclophosphamide, and rituximab.

A final option for patients with ongoing disease activity on mono-therapy with a standard agent is to add another agent. Although there is a seemingly strong rationale for such combination therapy in MS and a number of small studies have supported the tolerability and utility of this approach, larger trials have yielded disappointing or conflicting results [51,52]. The most common approaches to combina-tion are to add methotrexate, azathioprine, mycophenolate mofetil, or intermittent courses of intravenous methlyprednisolone to an IFN-β or glatiramer acetate.

Clinically isolated syndromes

Patients with a CIS and multiple MRI lesions are at high risk of devel-oping additional MRI or clinical events leading to the diagnosis of RR MS within several years [16]. All of the standard agents have been shown in randomized controlled trials to be effective in decreasing this risk [53–56]. Although it is not advisable to initiate disease therapy in every patient with a CIS, the possibility of MS and the pros and cons of initiating therapy need to be considered and discussed with all patients. Patients with a mild initial relapse with good recovery and no or only a few MRI lesions are at low risk and can be followed clinically and with periodic MRI. The following patients should be considered for therapy:

- patients with a severe initial relapse and/or with incomplete recovery;
- patients with more than two cranial MRI lesions characteristic of MS; or
- patients with evidence of intrathecal antibody production on CSF examination.

Patients with atypical clinical or imaging features require further diagnostic evaluation prior to making a decision. The patient's priorities also are an important factor in this decision.

Treatment of progressive multiple sclerosis

Progressive MS includes patients with SP MS (progression that develops after an initial RR course), primary progressive (PP) MS (progression from onset), and progressive-relapsing MS (progression from onset with subsequent superimposed relapses). There is increasing evidence that the three forms of progressive MS have similar pathogenesis in which degenerative processes predominate and the inflammatory activity most directly reflected by relapses and MRI lesion activity is less prominent [57].

As a result, immunomodulatory disease therapies tend to be less effective when the disease is purely progressive, and the evidence supporting efficacy of MS disease therapies in progressive MS is less robust than in RR MS. Randomized controlled trials have supported the efficacy of mitoxantrone in SP MS [28]. Some studies of IFN-β [58,59], but not others [60,61], have shown benefit. Trials in PP MS have been uniformly negative, although a subset of patients may have benefited from glatiramer acetate [62] or rituximab [63]. In general, the patients with progressive MS who are most likely to benefit from disease therapies are young, have had a short duration of progression, and have had recent relapses or MRI lesion activity.

In patients with progressive MS we feel it is reasonable to attempt therapy with the standard disease therapies glatiramer acetate or IFN-β, with the understanding that if these are ineffective or side effects outweigh benefit they should be discontinued. Other options include 3- to 5-day courses of intravenous methlyprednisolone repeated every 2 or 3 months, low-dose oral methotrexate, or intravenous Ig every 1 to 2 months, although the evidence for these approaches is largely anecdotal or based on small studies (Level III or IV evidence). It also is reasonable to consider fingolimod or natalizumab in selected patients; both are being tested in progressive MS. More potent therapies (eg, mitoxantrone, cyclophosphamide, or mycophenolate mofetil) are reserved for patients with rapid progression and MRI lesion activity for whom other options are not available.

Prior to initiating disease-modifying therapy in patients with progressive disease, it is advisable to obtain updated imaging studies to assess for the presence of active lesions. This assists in predicting the likelihood of benefit and, along with screening blood studies, in ruling out other treatable disease processes that could be contributing to progressive disability. In addition, health maintenance and rehabilitative approaches are of great importance.

Treatment of fulminant multiple sclerosis

Fulminant MS manifests as frequent severe relapses that recover incompletely with rapid accrual of disability or manifests as continued MRI lesion activity with rapid accumulation of lesions and atrophy progression. The long-term prognosis is poor. Standard disease therapies often are not sufficiently potent to control their disease. These patients are candidates for natalizumab or fingolimod, either as initial therapy or after a trial of first-line therapies. Other available strategies, described primarily in open-label studies or case reports (Level III or IV evidence) include cyclophosphamide induction therapy [64] and mycophenolate mofetil [65,66].

Multiple sclerosis treatment in children

MS presents before the age of 15 years in 3–5% of patients and rarely occurs in infancy or early childhood [67]. In nearly all children, MS begins with a RR course. The rationale for disease treatment is the same in early onset MS as for adults, to reduce relapses and MRI activity with the long-term goal of preventing permanent disability. Although none of the approved disease therapies has undergone definitive testing in children, limited experience supports glatiramer acetate and IFN-β in terms of efficacy, tolerability, and safety. Data on long-term safety are lacking. A recent systematic survey of the practice patterns of an expert panel of US physicians provided consensus on some specific treatment approaches, including the following [68]:

- intravenous methylprednisolone is the first-line treatment of choice for acute relapses of MS in children, although consensus was lacking regarding specific dose and treatment duration; and
- first-line disease-modifying therapies for pediatric MS were IFN-β and glatiramer acetate, chosen based on perceived efficacy and tolerability.

There was lack of agreement on the optimal choice of second-line treatments for acute relapses and a consensus was not reached on whether to use disease-modifying therapies in children under the age of 5 years, highlighting these as important areas for further study.

Devic's neuromyelitis optica

Historically, Devic's neuromyelitis optica (NMO) was viewed as a variant of MS, distinguished by epidemiologic, clinical, pathologic, imaging, prognostic, and therapeutic differences. NMO now is considered a distinct CNS inflammatory disorder [69]. Features that distinguish NMO from MS are summarized in Figure 5.3. A diagnostic serologic biomarker, NMO immunoglobulin G, is highly specific for NMO [70].

Features that distinguish Devic's neuromyelitis optica from multiple sclerosis

Like RR MS, acute relapses in NMO typically are treated with short courses of intravenous methylprednisolone followed by a tapering dose of oral prednisone. If the patient fails to respond, intravenous Ig or plasma exchanges are alternatives. Because NMO relapses often are severe, evolve rapidly, and recover incompletely, the threshold for early treatment is lower. Whereas treatment of MS relapses often is delayed initially when neurologic impairment is mild, in NMO it is advisable to begin treatment at the onset of periorbital neck/back pain when neurologic symptoms still may be mild.

NMO appears not to respond to approved standard disease therapies for MS. Although there are no definitive randomized controlled trials to provide guidance, typical initial disease therapy for NMO is a prolonged gradual tapering dose of oral corticosteroids with simultaneous initiation of azathioprine [71], aiming for a target dose that causes modest leukopenia and an increase in erythrocyte mean corpuscular volume (typically 2 or 3 mg/kg/day). This regimen is effective in approximately 50% of patients. Other options supported by small series (Level III or IV evidence) include mitoxantrone [72], rituximab [73,74], and mycophenolate mofetil [75].

Emerging anti-inflammatory therapies

A sizeable number of additional agents may soon be available to treat RR MS [76]. Agents that are currently in Phase III testing are listed in

Features that distinguish Devic's neuromyelitis optica from MS	
Clinical features	Recurrent episodes of optic neuritis or transverse myelitis that can be concurrent or sequential
	Symptomatic sparing of cerebrum
	Brainstem involvement when it occurs is by extension from the upper cervical spinal cord – often symptomatic
	Severe disability accumulation due to incomplete recovery from relapses rather than secondary progression
Pathologic features	Prominent perivascular accumulation of polymorphonuclear leukocytes, plasma cells, and eosinophils
	Hyaline changes in blood vessels
	Necrosis
Serologic features	Presence of NMO IgG (a highly specific, moderately sensitive marker for Devic's NMO)
Cranial MRI findings	Normal or scattered nonspecific T2 hyperintensities
	Medullary lesions, often contiguous extension from cervical cord
	Linear corpus callosum lesions
	Patchy hypothalamic, periventricular, periaqueductal lesions
Spine MRI findings	Homogeneous longitudinally extensive T2 signal abnormality
	Diffuse or patchy Gd-enhancement with cord enlargement during relapses
	Gd-enhancement can persist between relapses
	T1 hypointensity
	Spinal cord atrophy and/or cavitation

Figure 5.3 Features that distinguish Devic's neuromyelitis optica from MS.
Gd, gadolinium; IgG, immunoglobulin G; NMO, neuromyelitis optica.

Figures 5.4 and 5.5. In addition to these, a large number of other agents are in earlier stages of development. These medications vary in mechanisms of action, route of administration (including both oral and parenteral agents), potency, and safety. Thus, clinicians and patients will be faced with numerous choices and will have to balance convenience and potency versus tolerability and safety when selecting treatment.

Oral agents for multiple sclerosis

BG-12 is an oral formulation of dimethyl fumarate, an antipsoriatic agent with anti-inflammatory and neuroprotective properties [77]. Two Phase III studies of dimethyl fumarate in patients with RR MS were initiated in 2007: a dose of 240 mg twice a day and a dose of 240 mg three times a day are being investigated in the DEFINE and CONFIRM studies, the latter also including glatiramer acetate in a comparator arm. Preliminary results from the DEFINE trial were announced in 2011 and showed that BG-12 at 240 mg, either twice or three times a day, significantly reduced

Emerging oral agents for MS: disease therapies with positive Phase III trial results

Agent	Mechanism of action	Potential safety issues
Dimethyl fumarate (BG-12)	Immunomodulator	Hepatotoxicity
Teriflunomide	Dihydro-orotate dehydrogenase inhibitor (pyrimidine synthesis) Inhibits T and B cell proliferation	Pancytopenia, hepatotoxicity

Figure 5.4 Emerging oral agents for MS: disease therapies with positive Phase III trial results.

Emerging parenteral agents for MS: disease therapies in Phase III clinical trials

Agent	Mechanism of action	Potential safety issues
Alemtuzumab	Anti-CD52 MAb Depletes T and B cells	Lymphopenia, infection, Graves disease, ITP
Daclizumab	Anti-CD25 MAb IL-2R antagonist	Cutaneous reactions, infection, autoimmunity
Ocrelizumab	Anti-CD20 MAb	Systemic inflammatory response syndrome

Figure 5.5 Emerging parenteral agents for MS: disease therapies in Phase III clinical trials.
IL-2R, interleukin-2 receptor; ITP, idiopathic thrombocytopenia purpura; MAb, monoclonal antibody.

the proportion of patients with RR MS who experienced relapses at 2 years compared with placebo [78]. Significant reductions in relapse rate, disease activity on MRI scans, and in disability progression as detected by the Expanded Disability Status Scale (EDSS) were also noted. Data from the CONFIRM study supported these results, showing that the average number of MS relapses in a year was reduced versus placebo and glatiramer acetate [79]. Adverse events, including gastrointestinal side effects and facial flushing, are common at treatment onset but BG-12 is generally well tolerated. Importantly, the availability of long-term safety data from the use of BG-12 in the psoriasis setting distinguishes this agent from most of the other emerging MS therapies. A regulatory filing seeking approval of BG-12 for the treatment of MS was submitted to the FDA in February 2012.

Another oral agent with positive Phase III data in MS is teriflunomide, the active metabolite of leflunomide, an immunosuppressant effective in the treatment of autoimmune disorders, especially rheumatoid arthritis. Teriflunomide's main immunomodulatory effect is thought to be the inhibition of the biosynthesis of pyrimidine, a metabolic component crucial to the expansion and differentiation of T-lymphocytes [80]. In the Phase III TEMSO study, once-daily teriflunomide (7 mg or 14 mg) significantly reduced the annualized relapse rate compared with placebo in patients with RR MS [81]. The superiority of the drug versus placebo was confirmed for a range of MRI endpoints at both doses and disability progression (at the higher dose), and teriflunomide was generally well tolerated. Two further Phase III trials are investigating the efficacy and safety of 7 mg/day and 14 mg/day teriflunomide in RR MS compared to placebo (TOWER) or sub-cutaneous IFN-β-1a (TENERE). In addition, the TOPIC study is comparing the effect of teriflunomide 7 mg/day and 14 mg/day with placebo in the prevention of conversion to clinically definite MS in patients with CIS.

Preliminary Phase III results of the immunomodulator agent, laquinimod, showed modest efficacy in patients with RR MS [82,83]; further investigation is under consideration. Oral cladribine demonstrated efficacy in patients with RR MS in a Phase III study [84]; however, the drug did not receive regulatory approval in the USA and Europe, and its clinical development in MS has been halted.

Parenteral agents for multiple sclerosis

Several monoclonal antibody therapies are in late-stage clinical development for MS. Alemtuzumab is a humanized monoclonal antibody to CD52, a cell surface antigen present on all lymphocytes and monocytes. Intravenous administration of this drug leads to a rapid and long-lasting removal of lymphocyte populations from the circulation [85]. The 2-year CARE-MS-I Phase III trial compared alemtuzumab against IFN-β-1a in treatment-naive patients with early RR MS. Patients received two annual short cycles of 12 mg daily intravenous alemtuzumab, with infusions once a day for 5 consecutive days for the first treatment and then, a year later, three infusions during 3 consecutive days. Alemtuzumab significantly reduced the relapse rate over the course of 2 years, with a 55% reduction versus IFN-β-1a, but did not slow disease progression compared to IFN-β-1a [86]. No significant treatment differences on EDSS-based endpoints were noted. Alemtuzumab was generally well tolerated, with infusion-associated reactions most commonly observed. Preliminary results from the CARE-MS-II Phase III study in patients with RR MS who had experienced relapse while on a prior therapy were announced in 2011 and showed that alemtuzumab significantly reduced relapse rates and the worsening of disability over 2 years compared with IFN-β-1a [87].

Two additional monoclonal antibodies are currently undergoing Phase III evaluation in patients with RR MS. The efficacy and safety of daclizumab, a humanized monoclonal antibody directed against CD25 delivered via monthly injection under the skin, are being assessed in two Phase III studies. Similarly, two ongoing Phase III studies are currently investigating intravenous ocrelizumab, a humanized monoclonal antibody to CD20 (the antigen recognized by rituximab), in RR MS. This latter agent is also being evaluated in a Phase III study in patients with PP MS.

Neuroprotective therapies

In addition to anti-inflammatory treatment strategies, there is great need for neuroprotective and reparative strategies, particularly for progressive forms of MS. Potentially neuroprotective medications include minocycline, phenytoin, lamotrigine, lithium, flecainide, erythropoietin, and glutamate receptor antagonists. Potential repair-promoting strategies include medications (eg, glatiramer acetate and fingolimod), growth factors, and stem cells.

References

1 Dhib-Jalbut S. Mechanisms of action of interferons and glatiramer acetate in multiple sclerosis. *Neurology*. 2002;58(Suppl 4):S3-S9.

2 Bornstein MB, Miller A, Slagle S, et al. A pilot trial of Cop 1 in exacerbating-remitting multiple sclerosis. *N Engl J Med*. 1987;317:408-414.

3 Johnson KP, Brooks BR, Cohen JA, et al. Copolymer 1 reduces relapse rate and improves disability in relapsing–remitting multiple sclerosis: results of a phase III multicenter, double-blind, placebo-controlled trial. *Neurology*. 1995;45:1268-1276.

4 Comi G, Filippi M, Wolinsky JS, et al. European/Canadian multicenter, double-blind, randomized, placebo-controlled study of the effects of glatiramer acetate on magnetic resonance imaging-measured disease activity and burden in patients with relapsing multiple sclerosis. *Ann Neurol*. 2001;49:290-297.

5 Filippi M, Rovaris M, Rocca MA, et al. Glatiramer acetate reduces the proportion of new MS lesions evolving into "black holes". *Neurology*. 2001;57:731-733.

6 Comi G, Martinelli V, Rodegher M, et al. Effect of glatiramer acetate on conversion to clinically definite multiple sclerosis in patients with clinically isolated syndrome (PreCISe study): a randomised, double-blind, placebo-controlled trial. *Lancet*. 2009;374:1503-1511.

7 The IFNB Multiple Sclerosis Study Group. Interferon beta-1b is effective in relapsing–remitting multiple sclerosis. I. Clinical results of a multicenter, randomized, double-blind, placebo-controlled trial. *Neurology*. 1993;43:655-661.

8 Paty DW, Li DKB; the UBC MS/MRI Study Group. Interferon beta-1b is effective in relapsing–remitting multiple sclerosis. II. MRI analysis results of a multicenter, randomized, double-blind, placebo-controlled trial. *Neurology*. 1993;43:662-667.

9 IFNB Multiple Sclerosis Study Group, The University of British Columbia MS/MRI Analysis Group. Interferon beta-1b in the treatment of multiple sclerosis: final outcome of the randomized controlled trial. *Neurology*. 1995;45:1277-1285.

10 Jacobs LD, Cookfair DL, Rudick RA, et al. Intramuscular interferon beta-1a for disease progression in relapsing multiple sclerosis. *Ann Neurol*. 1996;39:285-294.

11 Rudick RA, Goodkin DE, Jacobs LD, et al. Impact of interferon beta-1a on neurologic disability in relapsing multiple sclerosis. *Neurology*. 1997;49:358-363.

12 Simon JH, Jacobs LD, Campion M, et al. Magnetic resonance studies of intramuscular interferon beta-1a for relapsing multiple sclerosis. *Ann Neurol*. 1998;43:79-87.

13 PRISMS Study Group. Randomized double-blind placebo-controlled study of interferon beta-1a in relapsing/remitting multiple sclerosis. *Lancet*. 1998;352:1498-1504.

14 Li DKB, Paty DW; the UBC MS/MRI Analysis Research Group, the PRISMS Study Group. Magnetic resonance imaging results of the PRISMS trial: a randomized, double-blind, placebo-controlled study of interferon-beta1a in relapsing–remitting multiple sclerosis. *Ann Neurol*. 1999;46:197-206.

15 PRISMS Study Group. PRISMS-4: long-term efficacy of interferon-beta-1a in relapsing MS. *Neurology*. 2001;56:1628-1636.

16 Ransohoff RM. Natalizumab for multiple sclerosis. *N Eng J Med*. 2007;356:2622-2629.

17 Polman CH, O'Connor PW, Hardova E, et al. A randomized, placebo-controlled trial of natalizumab for relapsing multiple sclerosis. *N Engl J Med*. 2006;354:899-910.

18 Miller DH, Soon D, Fernando KT, et al. MRI outcomes in a placebo-controlled trial of natalizumab in relapsing MS. *Neurology*. 2007;68:1390-1401.

19 Rudick RA, Stuart WH, Calabresi PA, et al. Natalizumab plus interferon beta-1a for relapsing multiple sclerosis. *N Engl J Med*. 2006;354:911-923.

20 Calabresi PA, Giovannoni G, Confavreux C, et al. The incidence and significance of anti-natalizumab antibodies. Results from AFFIRM and SENTINEL. *Neurology.* 2007;69:1391-1403.

21 Yousry TA, Major EO, Ryschkewitsch C, et al. Evaluation of patients treated with natalizumab for progressive multifocal leukoencephalopathy. *N Engl J Med.* 2006;354:924-933.

22 Khatri BO, Man S, Giaovannoni G, et al. Effect of plasma exchange in accelerating natalizumab clearance and restoring leukocyte function. *Neurology.* 2009;72:402-409.

23 Bozic C, Richman S, Plavina T, et al. Anti-John Cunnigham virus antibody prevalence in multiple sclerosis patients: Baseline results of STRATIFY-1. *Ann Neurol.* 2011;70:742-750.

24 Kappos L, Bates D, Hartung HP, et al. Natalizumab treatment for multiple sclerosis: recommendations for patient selection and monitoring. *Lancet Neurol.* 2007;6:431-441.

25 Millefiorini E, Gasperini C, Pozzilli C, et al. Randomized placebo-controlled trial of mitoxantrone in relapsing–remitting multiple sclerosis: 24-month clinical and MRI outcome. *J Neurol.* 1997;44:153-159.

26 Edan G, Miller D, Clanet M, et al. Therapeutic effect of mitoxantrone combined with methylprednisolone in multiple sclerosis: a randomised multicentre study of active disease using MRI and clinical criteria. *J Neurol Neurosurg Psychiatry.* 1997;62:112-118.

27 van de Wyngaeert FA, Beguin C, D'Hooghie MB, et al. A double-blind clinical trial of mitoxantrone versus methylprednisolone in relapsing, secondary progressive multiple sclerosis. *Acta Neurol Belg.* 2001;101:210-216.

28 Hartung HP, Gonsette R, the MIMS Study Group. Mitoxantrone in progressive multiple sclerosis: a placebo-controlled, randomised, multicentre trial. *Lancet.* 2002;360:2018-2025.

29 Krapf H, Morrissey SP, Zenker O, et al. Effect of mitoxantrone on MRI in progressive MS. Results of the MIMS trial. *Neurology.* 2005; 65:690-695.

30 Cohen BA, Mikol DD. Mitoxantrone treatment of multiple sclerosis. Safety considerations. *Neurology.* 2004;63(Suppl 6):S28-S32.

31 De Castro S, Cartoni D, Millefiorini E, et al. Noninvasive assessment of mitoxantrone cardiotoxicity in relapsing remitting multiple sclerosis. *J Clin Pharmacol.* 1995;35:627-632.

32 Ghalie RG, Edan G, Laurent M, et al. Cardiac adverse effects associated with mitoxantrone (Novantrone) therapy in patients with MS. *Neurology.* 2002;59:909-913.

33 Strotmann JM, Spindler M, Weilbach FX, et al. Myocardial function in patients with multiple sclerosis treated with low-dose mitoxantrone. *Am J Cardiol.* 2002;89:1222-1225.

34 Avasarala JR, Cross AH, Clifford DB, et al. Rapid onset mitoxantrone-induced cardiotoxicity in secondary progressive multiple sclerosis. *Mult Scler.* 2003;9:59-62.

35 Brassat D, Recher C, Waubant E, et al. Therapy-related acute myeloblastic leukemia after mitoxantrone treatment in a patient with MS. *Neurology.* 2002;59:954-955.

36 Ghalie RG, Mauch E, Edan G, et al. A study of therapy-related acute leukaemia after mitoxantrone therapy for multiple sclerosis. *Mult Scler.* 2002;8:441-445.

37 Cohen JA, Chun J. Mechanisms of fingolimod's efficacy and adverse effects in multiple sclerosis. *Ann Neurol.* 2011;69:759-777.

38 Kappos L, Radue EW, O'Connor P, et al. A placebo-controlled trial of oral fingolimod in relapsing multiple sclerosis. *N Engl J Med.* 2010;362:387-401.

39 Cohen JA, Barkhof F, Comi G, et al. Oral fingolimod or intramuscular interferon for relapsing multiple sclerosis. *N Engl J Med.* 2010;362:402-415.

40 Sorensen PS, Deisenhammer F, Dudac P, et al. Guidelines on use of anti-IFN-beta antibody measurements in multiple sclerosis: report of an EFNS Task Force on IFN-beta antibodies in multiple sclerosis. *Eur J Neurol.* 2005;12:817-827.

41 Goodin DS, Frohman EM, Garmany GP, et al. Disease modifying therapies in multiple sclerosis. Report of the Therapeutics and Technology Assessment Subcommittee of the American Academy of Neurology and the MS Council for Clinical Practice Guidelines. *Neurology.* 2002;58:169-178.

42 The Once Weekly Interferon for MS Study Group (OWIMS). Evidence of interferon beta-1a dose response in relapsing–remitting MS. The OWIMS study. *Neurology.* 1999;53:679-686.

43 Durelli L, Verdun E, Barbero P, et al. Every-other-day interferon beta-1b versus once-weekly interferon beta-1a for multiple sclerosis: results of a 2-year prospective randomized multicentre study (INCOMIN). *Lancet.* 2002;359:1453-1460.

44 Panitch H, Goodin DS, Francis G, et al. Randomized, comparative study of interferon b-1a treatment regimens in MS. The EVIDENCE trial. *Neurology.* 2002;59:1496-1506.

45 Schwid SR, Thorpe J, Sharief M, et al. Enhanced benefit of increasing interferon beta-1a dose and frequency in relapsing multiple sclerosis. The EVIDENCE study. *Arch Neurol.* 2005;62:785-792.

46 Clanet M, Radue EW, Kappos L, et al. A randomized, double-blind, dose-comparison study of weekly interferon beta-1a (Avonex) in relapsing MS. *Neurology.* 2002;59:1507-1517.

47 Goodin DS, Frohman EM, Hurwitz B, et al. Neutralizing antibodies to interferon beta: assessment of their clinical impact and radiographic impact: an evidence report. Report of the Therapeutics and Technology Assessment Subcommittee of the American Academy of Neurology. *Neurology.* 2007;68:977-984.

48 Mikol DD, Barkhof F, Chang P, et al. Comparison of subcutaneous beta-1a with glatiramer acetate in patients with relapsing multiple sclerosis (the REbif vs Glatiramer Acetate in Relapsing MS Disease [REGARD] study): a multicentre, randomised, parallel, open-label trial. *Lancet Neurol.* 2008;7:903-914.

49 O'Connor P, Filippi M, Arnason B, et al. 250 mg or 500 mg interferon beta-1b versus 20 mg glatiramer acetate in relapsing–remitting multiple sclerosis: a prospective, randomised, multicentre study. *Lancet Neurol.* 2009;8:889-897.

50 Rudick RA, Polman CH. Current approaches to the identification and management of breakthrough disease in patients with multiple sclerosis. *Lancet Neurol.* 2009;8:545-559.

51 Cohen JA, Imrey PB, Calabresi PA, et al. Results of the Avonex Combination Trial (ACT) in relapsing–remitting MS. *Neurology.* 2009;72:535-541.

52 Cohen JA, Confavreux C. Combination therapy in multiple sclerosis. In: Cohen JA, Rudick RA, eds. *Multiple Sclerosis Therapeutics*, *3rd Edition.* London, UK: Informa Healthcare; 2007:681-697.

53 Jacobs LD, Beck RW, Simon JH, et al. Intramuscular Interferon beta-1a therapy initiated during a first demyelinating event in multiple sclerosis. *N Engl J Med.* 2000;343:898-904.

54 Comi G, Filippi M, Barkhof F, et al. Effect of early interferon treatment on conversion to definite multiple sclerosis: a randomized study. *Lancet.* 2001;357:1576-1582.

55 Kappos L, Polman CH, Freedman MS, et al. Treatment with interferon beta-1b delays conversion to clinically definite and McDonald MS in patients with clinically isolated syndromes. *Neurology.* 2006;67:1242-1249.

56 Comi G, Martinelli V, Rodegher M, et al. Effect of glatiramer acetate on conversion to clinically definite multiple sclerosis in patients with clinically isolated syndrome (PreCISe study): a randomised, double-blind, placebo-controlled trial. *Lancet.* 2009;374:1503-1511.

57 Trapp BD, Nave K-A. Multiple sclerosis: an immune or neurodegenerative disorder? *Annu Rev Neurosci.* 2008;31:247-269.

58 Kappos L, Polman C, Pozzilli C, et al. Final analysis of the European multicenter trial on INFbeta-1b in secondary-progressive MS. *Neurology.* 2001;57:1969-1975.

59 Cohen JA, Cutter GR, Fischer JS, et al. Benefit of interferon beta-1a on MSFC progression in secondary progressive MS. *Neurology.* 2002;59:679-687.

60 The North American Study Group on Interferon Beta-1b in Secondary Progressive MS. Interferon beta-1b in secondary progressive MS: results from a three-year controlled study. *Neurology.* 2004;63:1788-1795.

61 Secondary Progressive Efficacy Clinical Trial of Recombinant Interferon-beta-1a in MS (SPECTRIMS) Study Group. Randomized controlled trial of interferon-beta-1a in secondary progressive MS. Clinical results. *Neurology.* 2001;56:1496-1504.

62 Wolinsky JS, Narayana PA, O'Connor P, et al. Glatiramer acetate in primary progressive multiple sclerosis: results of a multinational, multicenter, double-blind, placebo-controlled trial. *Ann Neurol.* 2007;61:14-24.

63 Hawker K, O'Connor P, Freedman MS, et al. Rituximab in patients with primary progressive multiple sclerosis. Results of a randomized double-blind placebo-controlled multicenter trial. *Ann Neurol.* 2009;66:460-471.

64 Smith DR, Weinstock-Guttman B, Cohen JA, et al. A randomized blinded trial of combination therapy with cyclophosphamide in patients with active multiple sclerosis on interferon beta. *Mult Scler.* 2005;11:573-582.

65 Ahrens N, Salama A, Haas J. Mycophenolate-mofetil in the treatment of refractory multiple sclerosis. *J Neurol.* 2001;248:713-714.

66 Frohman EM, Brannon K, Racke MK, et al. Mycophenolate mofetil in multiple sclerosis. *Clin Neuropharmacol.* 2004;27:80-83.

67 Ness JM, Chabas D, Sadovnick AD, et al. Clinical features of children and adolescents with multiple sclerosis. *Neurology.* 2007;68(Suppl 2):S37-S45.

68 Waldman AT, Gorman MP, Rensel MR, et al. Management of pediatric central nervous system demyelinating disorders: consensus of united states neurologists. *J Child Neurol.* 2011;26:675-682.

69 Weinshenker BG. Neuromyelitis optica is distinct from multiple sclerosis. *Arch Neurol.* 2007;64:899-901.

70 Lennon VA, Wingerchuk DM, Kryzer TJ, et al. A serum antibody marker of neuromyelitis optica: distinction from multiple sclerosis. *Lancet.* 2004;364:2106-2112.

71 Mandler RN, Ahmed W, Dencoff JE. Devic's neuromyelitis optica: a prospective study of seven patients treated with prednisone and azathioprine. *Neurology.* 1998;51:1219-1220.

72 Weinstock-Guttman B, Ramanathan M, Lincoff N, et al. Study of mitoxantrone for the treatment of recurrent neuromyelitis optica (Devic disease). *Arch Neurol.* 2006;63:957-963.

73 Cree BAC, Lamb S, Morgan K, et al. An open label study of the effects of rituximab in neuromyelitis optica. *Neurology.* 2005;64:1270-1272.

74 Jacob A, Weinshenker BG, Violich I, et al. Treatment of neuromyelitis optica with rituximab. Retrospective analysis of 25 patients. *Arch Neurol.* 2008;65:1443-1448.

75 Jacob A, Matiello M, Weinshenker BG, et al. Treatment of neuromyelitis optica with mycophenolate mofetil. *Arch Neurol.* 2009;66:1128-1133.

76 Cohen JA. Emerging therapies for relapsing multiple sclerosis. *Arch Neurol.* 2009;66:821-828.

77 Kappos L, Gold R, Miller DH, et al. Efficacy and safety of oral fumarate in patients with relapsing-remitting multiple sclerosis: a multicentre, randomised, double-blind, placebo-controlled phase IIb study. *Lancet.* 2008;372:1463-72.

78 Biogen Idec. Biogen Idec announces positive top-line results from the first phase 3 trial investigating oral BG-12 (DIMETHYL FUMARATE) in multiple sclerosis. www.biogenidec.com/press_release_details.aspx?ID=5981&ReqId=1548648. Accessed March 9, 2012.

79 Biogen Idec. Biogen Idec announces positive top-line results from second phase 3 trial investigating oral bg-12 (dimethyl fumarate) in multiple sclerosis. www.biogenidec.com/press_release_details.aspx?ID=5981&ReqId=1621631. Accessed March 9, 2012.

80 Tallantyre E, Evangelou N, Constantinescu CS. Spotlight on teriflunomide. *Int MS J.* 2008;15:62-68.

81 O'Connor P, Wolinsky JS, Confavreux C, et al. Randomized trial of oral teriflunomide for relapsing multiple sclerosis. *N Engl J Med.* 2011;365:1293-303.

82 Comi G. Oral laquinimod reduced relapse rate and delayed progression of disability in ALLEGRO, a placebo-controlled phase III trial for relapsing-remitting multiple sclerosis. *Neurology.* 2011;76(Suppl 4):7PP.001.

83 TevaPharma. Results of Phase III Bravo trial. www.tevapharm.com/en-US/Media/News/Pages/Bravo.aspx. Accessed March 9, 2012.

84 Giovannoni G, Comi G, Cook S, et al. A placebo-controlled trial of oral cladribine for relapsing multiple sclerosis. *N Engl J Med.* 2010;362:416-426.

85 Klotz L, Meuth SG, Wiendl H, et al. Immune mechanisms of new therapeutic strategies in multiple sclerosis- a focus on alemtuzumab. *Clin Immunol.* 2012;142:25-30.

86 Coles A, Brinar V, Arnold DL, et al. Efficacy and Safety Results from CARE-MS I: a Phase 3 study comparing alemtuzumab and interferon beta-1a. Abstract presented at ECTRIMS 2011.

87 Genzyme. Genzyme announces successful Phase III results for alemtuzumab in multiple sclerosis. www.businesswire.com/news/genzyme/20111113005072/en. Last updated November 14, 2011. Accessed March 9, 2012.

Chapter 6

Symptom management

General points

Multiple sclerosis (MS) potentially produces a wide variety of symptoms (see Figure 2.1), either during acute relapses or chronically. The combination of symptoms and their severity vary markedly from patient to patient and in individual patients over time. MS symptoms can interfere with daily activities or lessen quality of life (QOL), and many are amenable to treatment. Thus identification and treatment of symptoms is an important aspect of MS management.

General principles of MS symptom management are reviewed in [1,2] and summarized in Figure 6.1. With the exception of dalfampridine for the treatment of walking impairment, there are few definitive data confirming the efficacy of most symptomatic therapeutic strategies and even fewer data on comparative efficacy. Most of the recommendations made below are therefore based on Level III or IV evidence and many involve off label use of medications. The most frequently used medications are listed in Figure 6.2.

Impaired mobility

Impaired mobility is an important clinical hallmark of MS that can develop early in the disease process. Reduced mobility has been reported in up to 90% of individuals with MS and is a major cause of disability [3]. Approximately 50% of MS patients need some form of walking assistance within 15 years of disease onset [4,5]. Impaired mobility is particularly

J. A. Cohen and A. Rae-Grant, *Handbook of Multiple Sclerosis*,
DOI: 10.1007/978-1-907673-50-4_6, © Springer Healthcare 2012

General principles of symptom management in MS

Systematically review symptoms during visits; some symptoms must be actively sought

Symptoms evolve, so make symptom management an ongoing process

Prioritize those symptoms that are most disabling or have secondary complications

Set realistic treatment goals for symptom management

Address contributing factors and try nonpharmacologic approaches before starting drug therapy

When prescribing medications to treat symptoms:

- Start at a low dose and gradually increase the dose until therapeutic benefit is achieved or intolerable side effects develop

- If after an adequate trial, one medication is ineffective or cannot be tolerated, consider other medications

- Although monotherapy usually is preferable, combination therapy sometimes is more effective or may permit lower doses and better tolerability

- When possible, choose medications that can treat more than one symptom

- Remember that the goal is improved function and quality of life not maximum alleviation of neurologic signs

Consider adjunct therapies in addition to medications; eg, physical therapy to develop a stretching regimen for spasticity

Consider referral for diagnostic evaluation or specialized treatment for complex problems

For some symptoms, an alternative approach may be better than medication; eg, counselling for emotional distress in reaction to the recent diagnosis of MS

Some sequelae of MS cannot be treated with medications, such as family, employment, insurance issues

Figure 6.1 General principles of symptom management in MS.

important from the patient's perspective because it affects the ability to perform activities of daily living and has a substantial impact on overall QOL [3,6,7]. Furthermore, reduced mobility is associated with a high economic burden in individuals with MS arising from direct medical costs as well as indirect factors, such as impact on employment status through, for example, higher absenteeism rates due to impaired mobility [8–10]. Importantly, even mild levels of mobility impairment can impact function, QOL, and socioeconomic status [8].

In most patients, the cause of impaired mobility is multifactorial. Although defective motor control is the principal factor responsible for mobility impairment in MS, other contributory factors include visual impairment, vestibular symptoms, weakness, spasticity, ataxia, imbalance, sensory loss, pain, and fatigue. Effective management requires delineating the relative contributions of these factors. Referral to physical

Selected medications to treat symptoms of MS

Medications	Dose	Comments
Impaired mobility		
Dalfampridine	10 mg twice daily	
Oscillopsia		
Gabapentin	Initial: 100 mg 3 times daily or 300 mg at bedtime Maximum: 300–900 mg 3–4 times daily	
Ondansetron	8 mg twice daily	
Diazepam	2–10 mg 2–4 times daily	Sedating
Vertigo		
Meclizine	12.5–25.0 mg every 6–8 hours	Sedating
Scopolamine patch	Apply to skin every 3 days	
Ondansetron	8 mg twice daily	
Diazepam	2–10 mg 2–4 times daily	Sedating
Spasticity		
Baclofen	Initial: 10 mg 2–3 times daily Maximum: 20 mg 4 times daily, up to 120 mg in selected patients	May exacerbate weakness or ataxia
Tizanidine	Initial: 2–4 mg at bedtime Maximum: 32–36 mg/day in 3–4 doses	Less tendency to exacerbate weakness and ataxia compared to baclofen but more sedating
Gabapentin	Initial: 100 mg 3 times daily or 300 mg at bedtime Maximum: 300–900 mg 3–4 times daily	Useful as adjunct therapy, particularly for spasms or when there is coexisting neuropathic pain
Diazepam	2–10 mg 2–4 times daily	Sedating, useful as adjunct therapy for nocturnal spasms
Clonazepam	Initial: 0.5 mg at bedtime Maximum: 0.5–5 mg 1–3 times daily	Sedating, useful as adjunct therapy for nocturnal spasms
Dantrolene	25–100 mg 2–4 times daily	Least sedation but produces obligatory weakness
Botulinum toxin type A	Dose selected based on muscles affected, severity of muscle activity, prior response to treatment, and adverse event history Do not exceed a total dose of 360 units administered in a 3-month interval	

Figure 6.2 Selected medications to treat symptoms of MS (continues overleaf).

Selected medications to treat symptoms of MS (continued)

Medications	Dose	Comments
Nocturia		
Desmopressin acetate nasal spray	20 µg (0.2 mL) intranasally at bedtime	Combine with fluid restriction in the evening, monitor for hyponatremia
Detrusor hyperactivity		
Oxybutynin	2.5–5 mg 2–3 times daily	
Oxybutynin extended release	Initial: 5–10 mg once daily Maximum: 30 mg/day	
Tolterodine	1–2 mg twice daily	
Tolterodine long acting	2–4 mg/day	
Solifenacin succinate	Initial: 5 mg/day Maximum: 10 mg/day	
Trospium chloride	Initial: 20 mg/day Maximum: 20 mg twice daily	
Darifenacin	Initial: 7.5 mg/day Maximum: 15 mg/day	
Fesoterodine fumarate	Initial: 4 mg/day Maximum: 8 mg/day	
Flavoxate HCl	100–200 mg 3–4 times daily	
Botulinum toxin type A	Recommended total dose 200 units Do not exceed a total dose of 360 units administered in a 3-month interval	
Detrusor hyporeflexia		
Bethanechol	10–50 mg 2–4 times daily	Intermittent catheterization or urinary diversion often are preferable
Detrusor–sphincter dyssynergia		
Terazosin	5–10 mg at bedtime	When there is coexistent detrusor hyperactivity and detrusor–sphincter dyssynergia, anticholinergic medication can be combined with terazosin or intermittent catheterization
Constipation		
Bulk-forming agents		Combine with adequate fluid intake, dietary fiber, and exercise
Lactulose	1–4 tablespoons (15–60 mL) daily	

Figure 6.2 Selected medications to treat symptoms of MS (continues opposite).

Selected medications to treat symptoms of MS (continued)

Medications	Dose	Comments
Bowel urgency		
Bulk-forming agents		Combine with scheduled voiding, anticholinergic medications, or biofeedback
Erectile dysfunction		
Sildenafil citrate	50 mg 1 hour before sexual activity	Rule out other causes for sexual dysfunction
Tadalafil	5–20 mg 30 minutes prior to sexual activity or 2.5 mg/day	Rule out other causes for sexual dysfunction
Vardenafil	5–20 mg 1 hour prior to sexual activity	Rule out other causes for sexual dysfunction
Depression		
Selective serotonin reuptake inhibitors		In general, treatment of depression in MS is similar to other settings
Duloxetine HCl	Initial: 20 mg/day	
Amitriptyline or nortriptyline	See below	Useful when there is coexisting neuropathic pain, detrusor hyperactivity, or sleep disturbance
Fatigue		
Amantadine	Initial: 100 mg in the morning Maximum: 100 mg twice daily, three times daily in selected patients	The second dose should be in the early afternoon to avoid sleep disturbance
Modafinil	Initial: 50–100 mg in the morning Maximum: 100 mg twice daily	The second dose should be in the early afternoon to avoid sleep disturbance
Armodafinil	Initial: 150 mg in the morning Maximum: 250 mg in the morning	
Neuropathic pain		
Pregabalin	Initial: 50 mg 3 times daily Maximum: 100 mg 3 times daily	
Gabapentin	Initial: 100 mg 3 times daily or 300 mg at bedtime Maximum: 300–900 mg 3–4 times daily	
Duloxetine HCl	Initial: 20 mg/day Maximum: 20 mg 3 times daily 60 mg once daily	Useful when there is coexisting depression

Figure 6.2 Selected medications to treat symptoms of MS.

Selected medications to treat symptoms of MS (continued)

Medications	Dose	Comments
Neuropathic pain (continued)		
Amitriptyline	Initial: 25 mg at bedtime Maximum: 100–150 mg at bedtime	Sedating and anticholinergic effects may be helpful if there is coexisting sleep disturbance or detrusor hyperactivity, or may be dose limiting
Nortriptyline	Initial: 25 mg at bedtime Maximum: 100–150 mg at bedtime	Sedating and anticholinergic effects may be helpful if there is coexisting sleep disturbance or detrusor hyperactivity, or may be dose limiting
Carbamazepine extended release	Initial: 200 mg twice daily Maximum: 400–600 mg twice daily	
Oxcarbazepine	Initial: 300 mg twice daily Maximum: 600 mg twice daily	
Phenytoin	200–400 mg/day in 1–4 divided doses	
Levetiracetam	500 mg twice daily	
Topiramate	Initial: 25 mg at bedtime Maximum: 200 mg twice daily	

Figure 6.2 Selected medications to treat symptoms of MS (continued).

therapy may assist with this assessment and help in the development of an individualized gait and balance training program. Patients should be evaluated for the most appropriate assistive device, and the need for a power mobility device should be considered. Home assessment should be undertaken to confirm that the necessary adaptations are present; for instance, installing grab bars, shower chairs, and hand rails for stairs, and eliminating dangerous features, such as throw rugs. For nonambulatory patients, subsequent loss of ability to transfer independently also has important functional ramifications. Patients with severe leg weakness may utilize involuntary extensor tone to support their weight during transfers. In such instances, there may be a difficult trade-off between relieving painful spasms and preserving the ability to transfer. Physical and occupational therapy can assist by providing transfer strategies and assessing for assistive devices.

Although immunomodulatory therapies reduce relapse rate and magnetic resonance imaging (MRI)-associated disease activity, the benefits of these drugs on disease-specific symptoms, such as impaired mobility, have not been clearly established, highlighting the need for a pharmacological treatment that targets this specific symptom. Dalfampridine, a sustained-release formulation of 4-aminopyridine, was approved by the US Food and Drug Administration (FDA) in January 2010 as an oral medication to improve walking speed in patients with MS. 4-Aminopyridine is a broad-spectrum inhibitor of voltage-sensitive potassium channels that improves impulse conduction in demyelinated nerve fibers and increases synaptic transmitter release at nerve endings. Dalfampridine is administered as a 10-mg timed-release pill taken 12 hours apart on a daily basis and can be used in combination with disease-modifying agents.

Two randomized, controlled Phase III studies assessed the efficacy and safety of dalfampridine in patients with MS, with response to treatment primarily based on changes in walking ability, measured with the Timed 25-Foot Walk (T25FW) [11,12]. In the first Phase III study, patients with MS who had a T25FW time between 8 and 45 seconds and Expanded Disability Status Scale (EDSS) scores of 2.5–7.0 received 14 weeks of treatment with either dalfampridine or placebo. The proportion of timed walk responders (based on consistency of walking speed improvement) was higher in the dalfampridine group than in the placebo group (35% vs 8%; $P<0.0001$) [11]; a change in timed walk ability of 20% or more has been suggested as the threshold that indicates a meaningful change in function [13]. The benefit observed with dalfampridine was observed in all MS disease types (ie, relapse–remitting [RR], primary progressive [PP], secondary progressive [SP], or progressive-relapsing). Overall, dalfampridine-treated responders demonstrated an improvement in walking speed of 25% compared with 5% in the placebo group. In addition, results obtained using the 12-item Multiple Sclerosis Walking Scale (MSWS-12), a rating scale that evaluates the patients' perspectives on their walking impairment, confirmed the validity of the responder analysis in this study; timed walk responders reported significantly greater average improvement from baseline in MSWS-12 scores than nonresponders ($P=0.0002$). The second Phase III study supported these results, showing a significantly greater proportion of timed walk responders in the dalfampridine group relative to placebo (43% vs 9%; $P<0.001$) across all MS subtypes [12]. Dalfampridine has a generally favorable safety and tolerability profile. The most frequent side effects of dalfampridine observed across both Phase III studies included urinary tract infection, dizziness, insomnia, paresthesias, nausea, and back pain. Seizures are recognized to be a dose-dependent risk for dalfampridine and a risk evaluation program is in place to inform physicians and patients about seizure risk [14]. Dalfampridine is therefore contraindicated in patients with a history of seizures or epileptiform changes on electroencephalography. It also is contraindicated in patients with moderate-to-severe renal impairment (creatinine clearance 50 mL/min or less).

Diplopia and oscillopsia

Brainstem lesions involving oculomotor pathways can cause diplopia. Symptoms from an acute lesion are treated with corticosteroids, as for other MS relapses, and eye patching. Chronic, stable diplopia may be addressed by prisms or eye muscle surgery. Brainstem lesions, particularly involvement of vestibular or cerebellar pathways, also can cause nystagmus with resultant oscillopsia. In some cases, gabapentin, ondansetron, or benzodiazepines, such as diazepam, may be helpful.

Vertigo

Vertigo, a sense of movement of one's self or the environment, can result from MS lesions involving the central vestibular pathways or the cranial nerve VIII entry zone. Vertigo is the presenting symptom in approximately 5% of patients with MS, and occurs at some point in approximately 50%. Acute centrally mediated vertigo may be a manifestation of a brainstem relapse, and may respond to a short course of corticosteroids. Chronic residual vertigo may respond to meclizine, transdermal scopolamine patch, ondansetron, diazepam, or vestibular rehabilitation.

Other causes of vertigo, such as benign paroxysmal positional vertigo, Ménière's disease, cervicogenic vertigo, or migraine, should not be overlooked in patients with MS. In a review of 1153 patients with MS, benign paroxysmal positional vertigo was the etiology of new-onset vertigo in approximately 50% of patients and responded to Epley or Semont canalith repositioning maneuvers [15]. In patients with MS, nonvertiginous dizziness also can occur from medication-induced orthostatic hypotension (eg, from tizanidine).

Bulbar dysfunction

Patients with severe MS and significant dysarthria should be monitored for swallowing dysfunction and should undergo formal swallowing evaluation if there is a history of choking or aspiration pneumonia. When impaired swallowing is confirmed, altering food consistency may be helpful. When nutritional needs cannot be met safely with oral feeding, a feeding gastrostomy should be discussed.

Spasticity

Spasticity is defined as a velocity-dependent increase in tonic muscle stretch reflexes, resulting from damage to descending motor pathways. Clinically, spasticity is manifested as abnormally increased muscle tone, involuntary muscle spasms, and loss of motor function. Spasticity associated with weakness is a common feature of MS, reported in surveys by 50–70% of patients with approximately one-third reporting that spasticity affected daily activities [16,17].

Treatment of spasticity involves an integrated approach for which general practice guidelines have been published [18]. Patients can manage mild spasticity with routine daily stretching, for which they should receive initial instruction from a physical therapist. Patients with more severe spasticity require adjunctive medication, which should be titrated based on the complications of spasticity (ie, discomfort, impaired motor function, interference with positioning or hygiene, etc.) rather than solely on muscle tone noted on examination.

First-line medications for spasticity include baclofen, a γ-aminobutyric acid agonist, and tizanidine, an α_2-adrenergic agonist. Both medications reduce abnormal increased muscle tone and the frequency of muscle spasms in MS. Baclofen should be started at a low dose and gradually up-titrated to improve tolerability. The usual maximum dose is 80 mg/day but occasionally doses of 120 mg/day or more are tolerated and useful. Common side effects of baclofen include somnolence, confusion, and exacerbation of pre-existing weakness and ataxia. When high doses are administered, liver function should be monitored. Abrupt discontinuation of baclofen should be avoided, as it can produce seizures. Tizanidine has less tendency to exacerbate weakness and ataxia, compared with baclofen, but its most common dose-limiting side effects are sedation, dry mouth, edema, and orthostatic hypotension. To lessen these side effects, tizanidine also should be started at a low dose with gradual dose escalation. Some patients with severe spasticity benefit from baclofen and tizanidine in combination. Adjunctive medications that are sometimes useful for spasms include gabapentin and benzodiazepines. The most common side effect of both is sedation. Dantrolene typically is reserved for nonambulatory patients with severe spasticity who are sensitive to the sedating effects of other medications but are not affected by the muscle weakness it produces.

For patients with severe spasticity inadequately controlled by oral medications, intrathecal administration of baclofen using a programmable pump should be considered. Advantages include greater potency and fewer systemic side effects. Individualized, complex dosing regimens are possible. Potential complications include those related to:

- pump placement (eg, headache from spinal fluid leak, wound dehiscence, or infection);
- the pump itself (eg, pump or catheter malfunction, or infection); or
- medication (eg, weakness, sedation, or encephalopathy).

Typically, intrathecal baclofen is reserved for patients with severe spastic paraparesis who are no longer ambulatory, although some patients with severe spasticity out of proportion to weakness may benefit and maintain ambulatory ability.

One formulation of botulinum toxin type A, onabotulinumtoxin A, was approved by the FDA in 2010 for the treatment of upper-limb spasticity in disorders including MS. This approval followed several double-blind, placebo-controlled studies in which targeted intramuscular injections of onabotulinumtoxin A improved upper-limb spasticity after stroke [19]. After intramuscular injection, botulinum toxin inhibits acetylcholine release at the neuromuscular junction, reducing muscle contraction for 3–6 months. Botulinum toxin injection generally is safe and usually is straightforward, but localization with electromyography may be needed for small or deep muscles. Periodic reinjection is needed to maintain benefit. Botulinum toxin injection is most useful to treat spasticity affecting selected muscles, allowing preservation of function in other muscles and avoidance of systemic side effects. Botulinum toxin is generally considered as a second-line therapy for spasticity if oral agents fail. In bed-bound patients with severe lower extremity weakness and spasticity interfering with positioning and hygiene, chemical (eg, phenol) or surgical rhizotomy, tenotomy, or botulinum toxin can be helpful to improve range of motion, obviating the need for surgical placement of a baclofen pump placement and periodic refill.

Tremor

Tremor in MS is often associated with ataxia, and may include rest, postural, and action components. When severe, cerebellar tremor is extremely disabling and may prevent self care. Adaptive devices, including wrist weights, may help but are difficult to use if there is concomitant weakness. A variety of medications have been reported to reduce MS tremor, including isoniazid, glutethimide, primidone, gabapentin, levetiracetam, carbamazepine, ondansetron, oral tetrahydrocannabinol, clonazepam, and propranolol (all Level IV evidence). However, results generally have been disappointing in clinical practice. Stereotactic ablation of the ventrolateral thalamic nucleus or thalamic electrostimulation via implanted electrodes sometimes produces dramatic improvement, but it usually is self-limited [20]. Risks of surgical procedures include weakness, hemorrhage, and infection.

Bladder dysfunction

Bladder dysfunction affects up to 90% of patients with MS [16,17] and most often results from spinal cord involvement. Urinary symptoms affect daily activities, employment, social life, and QOL. Symptoms can result from failure to store urine (frequency, urgency, nocturia, and incontinence) or failure to empty (hesitancy and retention). Bladder dysfunction increases the risk for urinary tract infections, and conversely, urinary tract infections may worsen bladder symptoms and other MS manifestations.

Types of neurogenic bladder dysfunction include:

- detrusor hyperactivity, secondary to disinhibition of the detrusor reflex due to lesions in the descending autonomic pathways;
- detrusor hyporeflexia, secondary to interruption of the detrusor reflex circuit in the conus medullaris;
- outlet obstruction, due to detrusor–sphincter dyssynergia; or
- a combination of the above.

Appropriate therapy depends on the underlying pathophysiology. However, symptoms often are an inaccurate indication of the underlying pathophysiology. For example, frequency can result both from detrusor hyperactivity and from retention with overflow. Measuring post-void residual volume by catheterization or ultrasonography is a useful screening test; however, formal urologic evaluation, including urinalysis, urine culture, post-void residual measurement, urodynamic testing, renal ultrasound, and other upper tract imaging studies, is needed to rule out nonneurologic contributors to symptoms and to guide therapy, particularly in patients with mixed symptoms. Finally, it is important to remember that bladder manifestations evolve over time. Patients with initial detrusor hyperactivity often develop a mixed picture later. General practice guidelines for the evaluation and management of MS-related bladder dysfunction have been published [21].

Detrusor hyperactivity

The most common bladder disorder in MS is detrusor hyperactivity, which causes urinary frequency, urgency, nocturia, voiding of small urine volume, and, when severe, incontinence. Initial therapeutic approaches include decreasing or discontinuing diuretics, including medications, alcohol, and caffeine; timed voiding; and regulating fluid intake. If nocturia is the principal issue, fluid restriction in the evening or desmopressin acetate nasal spray at bedtime may be helpful. Hyponatremia is an occasional complication. Patients should be cautioned against treating urinary frequency by fluid restriction throughout the day: adequate urine flow is needed to prevent urinary tract infections and calculi, and lessen constipation. The primary treatment for detrusor hyperactivity is anticholinergic medication: oxybutynin, tolterodine, solifenacin succinate, trospium chloride, darifenacin, or fesoterodine. Extended-release and transdermal patch formulations often are better tolerated and more convenient. The main side effects of anticholinergic medications are dry mouth and constipation, and all of these agents are contraindicated in patients with narrow-angle glaucoma and asthma. Anticholinergics can exacerbate concomitant impaired bladder emptying, so when there is combined failure to store and to empty urine, anticholinergic medication plus intermittent or indwelling catheterization may be required. In 2011, onabotulinumtoxin A injection was FDA-approved for the treatment of urinary incontinence due to detrusor hyperactivity in people with neurologic conditions, such as MS or spinal cord injury. The treatment consists of botulinum toxin being injected into the bladder, resulting in relaxation of the bladder, an increase in its storage capacity and a decrease in urinary incontinence. In two randomized, placebo-controlled Phase III studies, the weekly frequency of incontinence episodes showed statistically significant decreases in patients receiving onabotulinumtoxin A compared with placebo [22,23]. The most common adverse events included urinary tract infection and urinary retention.

Detrusor hyporeflexia

Detrusor hyporeflexia leads to inadequate bladder contraction and resultant impaired emptying, urinary hesitancy, retention, and overflow incontinence, sometimes manifesting as frequency. Complications include urinary tract infections, bladder stones, and rarely hydronephrosis and renal failure. Sometimes suprapubic pressure (Credé's maneuver) or cholinergic agonists, such as bethanechol, are helpful to augment micturition, but most often urinary drainage is necessary. Intermittent catheterization by the patient or a caregiver is the preferred approach. When intermittent catheterization is not feasible, urinary diversion with an indwelling catheter is needed. Long-term urethral catheterization generally should be avoided due to the risk of infection and urethral dilation with resultant leakage. Suprapubic or other permanent catheters have less risk of these complications but require a surgical procedure.

Detrusor–sphincter dyssynergia

Detrusor–sphincter dyssynergia, failure of the urinary sphincter to relax during micturition, causes hesitancy, intermittent stream, impaired bladder emptying, retention, and sometimes overflow incontinence. Terazosin, an α_1-adrenergic antagonist, or sphincter injection with botulinum toxin sometimes are useful, but often intermittent self-catheterization is the most effective therapy. Detrusor–sphincter dyssynergia often occurs in combination with detrusor hyperactivity, leading to mixed symptoms and complicating therapy. In this setting both components must be treated.

Future directions for treatment

Electrical bladder or sacral root stimulation recently has shown promise in the treatment of a variety of urinary symptoms. However, at present, this approach precludes MRI, limiting its utility in MS.

Bowel dysfunction

Approximately two-thirds of patients with MS report bowel dysfunction [16,17]. The most common symptom is constipation, which often has multiple contributing factors, including loss of autonomic input to the gut, side effects of anticholinergic and other medications, fluid restriction, inadequate dietary intake of fiber, and decreased mobility. Management of chronic constipation includes patient and caregiver education, addressing contributing factors, maintaining adequate fluid and fiber intake, bulk-forming agents, such as psyllium or methylcellulose, stool softeners (eg, docusate sodium), scheduled defecation, and increasing physical activity. When a laxative is needed, lactulose is useful. Chronic use of stimulants should be avoided. Some patients have diarrhea and incontinence either as a primary symptom or secondary to constipation (ie, leakage around retained stool). Anticholinergic medications and biofeedback are helpful for fecal urgency and incontinence.

Sexual dysfunction

Sexual dysfunction occurs in up to 75% of patients with MS [16,17]. Its frequency often is underestimated because patients, significant others, and clinicians may feel uncomfortable discussing it. Contributing factors include direct neurogenic effects, indirect effects of other MS symptoms (eg, decreased sensation, spasticity, incontinence, or pain), depression, marital relationship problems, and side effects of medications, such as decreased libido from antidepressants or vaginal dryness from anticholinergics. Men report decreased libido, erectile dysfunction, and delayed ejaculation. Women report decreased libido, anorgasmia, and dyspareunia. Both may report decreased genital sensation.

Management should involve the neurologic team, a urologist with expertise in sexual dysfunction or a sex therapist, the patient, and the partner. Education and counselling are useful in both sexes. Oral phosphodiesterase-5 inhibitors – sildenafil, tadalafil, and vardenafil – improve male erectile dysfunction. Other options include vibratory stimulation, vacuum pumps, papaverine or prostaglandin E_1 injections, and implanted penile prostheses, but these have been largely supplanted by the phosphodiesterase-5 inhibitors. Pharmacologic treatment options for female sexual dysfunction are more limited. No medication has demonstrated benefit for female anorgasmia. The management of other contributing symptoms (eg, lubrication), vibratory stimulation, and adequate sexual positioning, can be helpful.

Cognitive impairment

Approximately 50% of patients with MS develop significant cognitive impairment, sometimes early in the disease or out of proportion to physical manifestations [24,25]. The most common deficits are in sustained attention, information-processing speed, working memory, verbal and visuospatial memory, and executive functions. Symptoms include forgetfulness, distractibility, difficulty multitasking, or "cognitive fatigue". Cognitive impairment should be considered in patients who appear to be struggling in social or work activities more than can be accounted for by their physical impairment.

Impairment may not be apparent during standard interview and bedside testing in the office. Although several screening tools have been reported, formal neuropsychological testing is needed to accurately diagnose, qualitatively characterize, and quantify the severity of cognitive deficits in MS.

Management includes educating (and often reassuring) the patient and family about the specific deficits. Contributing factors should be addressed, including depression, fatigue, sleep disorders, and medication side effects. Compensatory strategies, such as pacing, memory aides, and environmental adaptations, often can be developed. Cognitive rehabilitation strategies are beginning to be explored in MS. Acetylcholinesterase inhibitors that are used to treat Alzheimer's disease, such as donepezil or memantine, are only occasionally helpful and not approved by regulatory agencies for use in MS. A recent study reported worsening MS symptoms with higher doses of memantine [26].

Mood disorders

Several studies have shown that depression and suicide are increased in MS [27–30]. Because MS, which is often disabling and unpredictable, typically presents in young adults who are starting their careers and families, depression may be reactive. However, the frequency of depression in MS is higher than most other chronic diseases, suggesting that organic causes related to the disease process or its treatment are involved. High-dose corticosteroids used to treat MS relapses can induce mood disorders both during therapy and with discontinuation [31]. The initial Phase III study of interferon-beta-1b (IFN-β-1b) in RR MS implicated IFNs in worsening MS-associated depression [32]. However, subsequent studies of all of the IFN-β agents in RR and SP MS did not support this association. Because of the high prevalence and sometimes serious consequences of depression in MS, it is important for clinicians to actively screen for it during office visits. Symptoms of depression can be confused with MS-related fatigue, cognitive impairment, or medication side effects.

Treatment of MS-related depression is similar to that in other settings. A combination of antidepressant medication and supportive psychotherapy is advisable in most patients. Referral to psychiatry should be considered if there are severe psychiatric issues (eg, psychosis, bipolar affective disorder, or substance abuse) or if initial medications are not effective. Selective serotonin reuptake inhibitors are first-line medications for depression in patients with MS. The specific medication choice is based on side-effect profiles, drug interactions, and other symptoms for which treatment is sought. In patients with coexisting neuropathic pain, duloxetine or tricyclics may be useful. Similarly, the anticholinergic effects of tricyclics may be useful when there is concomitant detrusor hyperactivity.

Pseudobulbar affect, also known as affective lability or emotional incontinence, can occur in MS and may be disconcerting to the patient or family; it is characterized by sudden, uncontrollable outbursts of laughter or crying, which is not a reflection of present mood. These can be triggered by external stimuli or be spontaneous. It responds to selective serotonin inhibitors, tricyclic antidepressants, or a recently tested dextromethorphan/quinidine combination. A combination of dextromethorphan hydrobromide (a potent σ-1 receptor agonist that suppresses excitatory neurotransmitter release) and quinidine sulfate (antagonizes the metabolism of dextromethorphan, raising circulating levels) has been shown in multiple Phase III studies to reduce the frequency of these outbursts while improving QOL measures in MS patients [33,34]. Present dosing consists of a mixture of 20 mg of dextromethorphan hydrobromide and 10 mg of quinidine sulfate twice a day in a fixed dosing schedule. When taking such prescribed dosing, the following should be avoided: antidepressants (due to an increased risk of serotonin syndrome), monoamine oxidase inhibitors, anticoagulants, over-the-counter dextromethorphan and quinidine products, and in patients with electrocardiographic abnormalities.

Fatigue

Fatigue is one of the most commonly disabling symptoms of MS but remains poorly understood. To date, studies have failed to demonstrate a clear-cut relationship between MS-related fatigue and physical impairment or MRI findings. Several types of MS-related fatigue exist:

- Handicap fatigue: tiring related to increased work of carrying out tasks due to neurologic impairment.
- Motor fatigue: worsening of pre-existing neurologic manifestations with exertion.

- Heat intolerance: accentuation of symptoms with increased body temperature analogous to Uthoff's phenomenon.
- Systemic fatigue: a persistent sense of lassitude unrelated to the above factors – probably the least well understood type of MS-related fatigue.

A number of other factors can contribute to fatigue in patients with MS. Other disorders that cause fatigue include thyroid disease, anemia, diabetes, vitamin B_{12} deficiency, and depression. Disturbed sleep is common due to nocturia, spasms, uncomfortable sensory symptoms, and obstructive sleep apnea. Many medications used in MS produce fatigue and somnolence as side effects. Thus, fatigue in patients with MS is best managed with a multidisciplinary approach, as outlined in published general practice guidelines [35].

The initial treatment approach should focus on addressing contributing factors, energy conservation, work simplification, and heat management strategies. An aerobic exercise program to gradually increase endurance should be undertaken, with the guidance of a physical therapist or trainer if needed. When medication is needed, amantadine, modafinil, and armodafinil are appropriate first-line agents, though none has regulatory approval for MS fatigue. The first dose should be taken in the morning; if a second dose is needed, it should be taken in the early afternoon to avoid causing insomnia at night. Patients on amantadine should be monitored for livedo reticularis. Patients on modafinil or armodafinil should be monitored for hypertension, headache, and weight loss. A small study reported benefit of aspirin for MS fatigue [36]. Amphetamine/dextroamphetamine, methylphenidate, and fluoxetine are helpful in some patients. All of these agents sometimes cause insomnia or a "jittery" feeling rather than a beneficial increase in energy.

Positive sensory phenomena and pain

Although its prevalence varies greatly between studies, pain is common in patients with MS [16,17]. It arises via several mechanisms.

Paroxysmal positive sensory phenomenon represent spontaneous nerve impulse generation in sensory pathways, induced by mechanical stretch of the cervical cord, such as Lhermitte's phenomenon, or sensory stimulation on the face (eg, trigeminal neuralgia). Rarely, demyelinated lesions develop in the entry zone of other cranial nerves or spinal roots, producing, for example, glossopharyngeal neuralgia or pseudo-radiculopathy, respectively. The resultant positive sensory phenomena can range from mild paresthesias to severe sharp electric shock-like pain. Medication options include carbamazepine, phenytoin, pregabalin, gabapentin, tiagabine, levetiracetam, topiramate, duloxetine, or tricyclic antidepressants. Severe trigeminal neuralgia that is not controllable by medication may respond to ablation of the trigeminal ganglion by balloon compression, glycerol, or gamma knife or nerve root section in the posterior fossa.

Demyelinated lesions in sensory pathways, particularly in the spinal cord, with resultant complex central nervous system remodeling and sensitization can result in chronic paresthesias, dysesthesias, or pain syndromes. These lesions most often involve the lower extremities but in some patients also involve the arms, trunk, or face. Medication options are similar to those used for neuralgic pain. In severe cases, oral narcotic analgesics, intrathecal analgesics, or spinal cord stimulation may be needed, in collaboration with a pain management specialist. Medical/surgical management should be combined with other approaches, such as biofeedback or acupuncture.

Pain also can result from a number of secondary complications of MS. Treatment is dictated by the cause. Optic neuritis and transverse myelitis often are accompanied by localized pain at the onset, due to irritation of adjacent meninges. This type of MS pain typically responds to corticosteroid treatment of the relapse. Patients with severe spasticity may experience painful spasms. Treatment approaches are the same as for other manifestations of spasticity. Back, neck, and upper and lower extremity pain of musculoskeletal origin are commonly encountered in the general population. In MS, trunk and limb weakness, abnormal posture, gait impairment, or tremor can lead to accelerated degenerative arthritis, particularly of the shoulders, neck, lumbar spine, hips, and knees. This issue should not be neglected because it represents a source of added disability, discomfort, and medical complications.

Some studies have shown a higher prevalence of headaches among patients with MS than among controls. Since patients with MS often take multiple medications, headache might be related to drug side effects. For example, IFN-β can exacerbate headaches in patients with a pre-existing migraine syndrome.

References

1   Goldman MD, Cohen JA, Fox RJ, et al. Multiple sclerosis: treating symptoms and other general medical issues. *Cleve Clin J Med.* 2006;73:177-186.

2   Boissy AR, Cohen JA. Multiple sclerosis symptom treatment. *Expert Rev Neurother.* 2007;7:1213-1222.

3   Hemmett L, Holmes J, Barnes M, et al. What drives quality of life in multiple sclerosis? *Q J Med.* 2004;97:671-676.

4   Weinshenker BG, Bass B, Rice GP, et al. The natural history of multiple sclerosis: a geographically based study. I. Clinical course and disability. *Brain.* 1989;112:133-146.

5   Myhr KM, Riise T, Vedeler C, et al. Disability and prognosis in multiple sclerosis: demographic and clinical variables important for the ability to walk and awarding of disability pension. *Mult Scler.* 2001;7:59-65.

6   Paltamaa J, Sarasoja T, Leskinen E, et al. Measures of physical functioning predict self-reported performance in self-care, mobility, and domestic life in ambulatory persons with multiple sclerosis. *Arch Phys Med Rehabil.* 2007;88:1649-1657.

7   Wu N, Minden SL, Hoaglin DC, et al. Quality of life in people with multiple sclerosis: data from the Sonya Slifka Longitudinal Multiple Sclerosis Study. *J Health Hum Serv Adm.* 2007;30:233-267.

8   Salter AR, Cutter GR, Tyry T, et al. Impact of loss of mobility on instrumental activities of daily living and socioeconomic status in patients with MS. *Curr Med Res Opin.* 2010;26:493-500.

9   Patwardhan MB, Matchar DB, Samsa GP, et al. Cost of multiple sclerosis by level of disability: a review of literature. *Mult Scler.* 2005;11:232-239.

10 Moreau R, Salter AR, Tyry T, et al. Work absenteeism and mobility levels in the NARCOMS registry. Poster S95 presented at the 24th Annual Meeting of the Consortium of Multiple Sclerosis Centers, June 2-5, 2010, San Antonio, Texas.

11 Goodman AD, Brown TR, Krupp LB, et al. Sustained-release oral fampridine in multiple sclerosis: a randomised, double-blind, controlled trial. *Lancet.* 2009;373:732-738.

12 Goodman AD, Brown TR, Edwards KR, et al. A Phase 3 trial of extended release oral dalfampridine in multiple sclerosis. *Ann Neurol.* 2010;68:494-502.

13 Schwid SR, Goodman AD, McDermott MP, et al. Quantitative functional measures in MS: what is a reliable change? *Neurology.* 2002;58:1294-1296.

14 Ampyra (dalfampridine) extended release tablets. *Risk evaluation and mitigation strategy.* www.accessdata.fda.gov/drugsatfda_docs/label/2010/022250s000REMS.pdf. Accessed March 9, 2012.

15 Frohman EM, Zhang H, Dewey RB, et al. Vertigo in MS: utility of positional and particle repositioning maneuvers. *Neurology.* 2000;55:1566-1568.

16 Poser S, Wikstrom J, Bauer HJ. Clinical data and the identification of special forms of multiple sclerosis in 1271 cases studied with a standardized documentation system. *J Neurol Sci.* 1979;40:159-168.

17 Goodin DS. Survey of multiple sclerosis in northern California. *Mult Scler.* 1999;5:77-88.

18 Haselkorn JK, Balsdon Richer C, Fry-Welch D, et al. Multiple Sclerosis Council for Clinical Practice Guidelines: spasticity management in multiple sclerosis. *J Spinal Cord Med.* 2005;28:167-199.

19 Yablon SA, Brin MF, VanDenburgh AM, et al. Dose response with onabotulinumtoxinA for post-stroke spasticity: a pooled data analysis. *Mov Disord.* 2011;26:209-215.

20 Montgomery EB, Baker KB, Kinkel RP, et al. Chronic thalamic stimulation for the tremor of multiple sclerosis. *Neurology.* 1999;53:625-628.

21 Seland TP, Brunette J, Clesson IM, et al. *Clinical Practice Guidelines: Urinary Dysfunction and Multiple Sclerosis.* Multiple Sclerosis Council for Clinical Practice Guidelines, 1999. Consortium for MS Centers. mscare.org/cmsc/index.php. Accessed March 9, 2012.

22 Cruz F, Herschorn S, Aliotta P, et al. Efficacy and safety of onabotulinumtoxinA in patients with urinary incontinence due to neurogenic detrusor overactivity: a randomised, double-blind, placebo-controlled trial. *Eur Urol.* 2011;60:742-750.

23 Ginsberg D, Gousse A, Keppenne V, et al. Phase 3 efficacy and safety study of onabotulinumtoxina in patients with urinary incontinence due to neurogenic detrusor overactivity. Abstract presented at the American Urological Association annual meeting 2011; abstract 1515.

24 Rao SM, Leo GJ, Bernardin L, et al. Cognitive dysfunction in multiple sclerosis. I. Frequency, patterns, and prediction. *Neurology.* 1991;41:685-691.

25 Rao SM, Leo GJ, Ellington L, et al. Cognitive dysfunction in multiple sclerosis. II. Impact on employment and social functioning. *Neurology.* 1991;41:692-696.

26 Villoslada P, Arrondo G, Sepulcre J, et al. Memantine induces reversible neurologic impairment in patients with MS. *Neurology.* 2009;72:1630-1633.

27 Sadovnick A, Eisen K, Ebers GC, et al. Cause of death in patients attending multiple sclerosis clinics. *Neurology.* 1991;41:1193-1196.

28 Sadovnick AD, Remick RA, Allen J, et al. Depression and multiple sclerosis. *Neurology.* 1996;46:628-632.

29 Feinstein A. An examination of suicidal intent in patients with multiple sclerosis. *Neurology.* 2002;59:674-678.

30 Edwards L, Constantinescu C. A prospective study of conditions associated with multiple sclerosis in a cohort of 658 consecutive outpatients attending a multiple sclerosis center. *Mult Scler.* 2004;10:575-581.

31 Wada K, Yamada N, Sato T, et al. Corticosteroid-induced psychotic and mood disorders: diagnosis defined by DSM-IV and clinical pictures. *Psychosomatics.* 2001;42:461-466.

32 The IFNB Multiple Sclerosis Study Group. Interferon beta-1b is effective in relapsing–remitting multiple sclerosis. I. Clinical results of a multicenter, randomized, double-blind, placebo-controlled trial. *Neurology.* 1993;43:655-661.

33 Panitch HS, Thisted RA, Smith RA, et al. Randomized, controlled trial of dextromethorphan/quinidine for pseudobulbar affect in multiple sclerosis. *Ann Neurol.* 2006;59:780-787.

34 Pioro EP, Brooks BR, Cumming J, et al. Dextromethorphan plus ultra low-dose quinidine reduces pseudobulbar affect. *Ann Neurol.* 2010;68:693-702.

35 Kinkel RP, Conway K, Copperman L, et al. *Clinical Practice Guidelines: Fatigue and Multiple Sclerosis. Multiple Sclerosis* Council for Clinical Practice Guidelines, 1998. Consortium of MS Centers. mscare.org/cmsc/index.php. Accessed March 9, 2012.

36 Wingerchuk DM, Benarroch EE, O'Brien PC, et al. A randomized controlled crossover trial of aspirin for fatigue in multiple sclerosis. *Neurology.* 2005;64:1267-1269.

Medical management of patients with multiple sclerosis

Health maintenance

The symptoms of multiple sclerosis (MS) overlap with those of a variety of medical conditions. Therefore, clinicians need to remain vigilant so as not to miss development of a coexisting disorder, which can cause fatigue (eg, anemia, thyroid disease, diabetes, or vitamin B_{12} deficiency) or a myelopathy (eg, cervical spondylosis). Patients with MS are predisposed to certain conditions, particularly decreased bone mineral density and vitamin D deficiency [1,2]. Furthermore, the adverse effects of some MS therapies increase the risk of certain conditions; for example, corticosteroids used to treat relapses can precipitate or exacerbate hyperglycemia, hypertension, or mood disorders. Although occasional courses of corticosteroids probably do not have deleterious effects on bone mineral density [3], chronic steroids may worsen bone mineral density loss. Chronic immunosuppression increases the risk of infection and malignancy. Finally, many MS disease therapies and symptomatic medications can cause drug-induced hepatitis.

Immunizations

In general, the indications for immunizations in patients with MS are the same as in the general population. Disabled patients with respiratory compromise or who are wheelchair- or bed-restricted should receive influenza and pneumococcal vaccinations. Prior to starting chronic

J. A. Cohen and A. Rae-Grant, *Handbook of Multiple Sclerosis*,
DOI: 10.1007/978-1-907673-50-4_7, © Springer Healthcare 2012

immunosuppressive therapy, it is advisable to consider vaccinating patients who do not have a history of chickenpox and/or have negative herpes zoster titers against shingles. In general, immunizations are safe and effective in patients with MS. Although there is a theoretical concern that immunizations could precipitate an MS relapse, in practice there is no convincing evidence of this [4]. Patients on chronic immunosuppression should not receive live-attenuated vaccines.

Sleep

Sleep disturbances are common in MS [5]. There are a number of potential causes related to MS, including pain, spasms, nocturia, depression, anxiety, restless leg syndrome, and obstructive sleep apnea. Chronic sleep deprivation can contribute to fatigue and cognitive impairment.

Smoking

In addition to its well-recognized deleterious effects on general health, smoking has been implicated as a risk factor for MS, independent of other environmental and genetic factors [6]. This observation further underscores the importance of assisting patients with smoking cessation.

Reproductive health

Because MS is more common in women and typically presents in early adulthood, reproductive issues commonly arise. In general, gynecologic care for women with MS is similar to that in the general population, but there are several special issues. Long-term immunosuppressive therapy potentially increases the risk of cervical neoplasms, so routine gynecologic examinations are important for women receiving these therapies. Mitoxantrone, cyclophosphamide, and rarely interferon-beta (IFN-β) cause menstrual irregularity or amenorrhea, particularly in premenopausal women. Women must be advised of this risk before initiating these therapies.

MS does not affect fertility. In the PRIMS study, a large prospective study of pregnancy in MS [7], there was no apparent increase in congenital abnormalities or complications of pregnancy, labor, or delivery. However, there may be a higher incidence of babies who are small for gestational age [8]. In general, no special precautions or measures are needed during pregnancy, labor, or delivery, including with anesthesia. The principal consideration is that disease therapies and most symptomatic medications should be avoided by women trying to conceive, during pregnancy, and while breastfeeding. At the Mellen Center, women are typically advised to discontinue IFN-β and glatiramer acetate 1 month and natalizumab and immunosuppressants 3 months prior to trying to become pregnant. The PRIMS study confirmed previous reports that the relapse rate tends to decrease during pregnancy but increases for 3–6 months post partum [7]. In general, at the Mellen Center we have a somewhat higher threshold for treating relapses that occur during pregnancy, particularly in the first trimester. However, if needed, relapses in pregnancy can be treated using the standard regimen, in collaboration with the patient's obstetrician.

Disease-modifying therapy should be restarted early after delivery in women with previously active disease. These therapies are not recommended while breastfeeding. In most cases, therapy can be deferred if the woman prefers to breastfeed. Some studies suggest that breastfeeding may lessen relapse risk [9].

Multidisciplinary care

MS potentially causes a wide variety of neurologic symptoms, medical complications, and psychosocial sequelae that vary both between patients and in individual patients over time. This complex disorder is best managed using a multidisciplinary team approach that includes neurology, nursing/physician assistants, clinical and cognitive psychology, physical therapy, occupational therapy, speech therapy, social work, and other medical specialties (physical medicine and rehabilitation, psychiatry, urology, neuro-ophthalmology, pain management, and internal medicine/primary care).

References

1   Nieves JW, Cosman F, Herbert J, et al. High prevalence of vitamin D deficiency and reduced bone mass in multiple sclerosis. *Neurology.* 1994;44:1687-1692.

2   Cosman F, Nieves J, Komar L, et al. Fracture history and bone loss in patients with MS. *Neurology.* 1998;51:1161-1165.

3 Schwid SR, Goodman AD, Puzas JE, et al. Sporadic corticosteroid pulses and osteoporosis in multiple sclerosis. *Arch Neurol.* 1996;53:753-757.

4 Miller AE, Morgante LA, Buchwald LY, et al. A multicenter, randomized, double-blind, placebo-controlled trial of influenza immunization in multiple sclerosis. *Neurology.* 1997;48:312-314.

5 Tachibana N, Howard RS, Hirsch NP, et al. Sleep problems in multiple sclerosis. *Eur Neurol.* 1994;34:320-323.

6 Riise T, Nortvedt MW, Ascherio A. Smoking is a risk factor for multiple sclerosis. *Neurology.* 2003;61:1122-1124.

7 Confavreux C, Hutchinson M, Hours MM, et al. Rate of pregnancy-related relapse in multiple sclerosis. *N Engl J Med.* 1998;339:285-291.

8 Dahl J, Myhr K-M, Daltveit AK, et al. Pregnancy, delivery, and birth outcome in women with multiple sclerosis. *Neurology.* 2005;65:1961-1963.

9 Langer-Gould A, Huang SM, Gupta R, et al. Exclusive breastfeeding and the risk of postpartum relapses in women with multiple sclerosis. *Arch Neurol.* 2009;66:958-963.

Resources

Books

Cohen JA and Rudick RA (eds). *Multiple Sclerosis Therapeutics, 4th Edition.*
New York, NY: Cambridge University Press; 2011.

Hill BA. *Multiple Sclerosis Q&A.* New York, NY: Avery; 2003.

Holland NJ, Murray TJ, Reingold SC. *Multiple Sclerosis, A Guide for the
Newly Diagnosed, 3rd edition.* New York, NY: Demos; 2007.

Compston A, Confavreux C, Lassman H, et al. *McAlpine's Multiple Sclerosis,
4th edition.* London, UK: Churchill Livingstone; 2005.

General information and best practices

American Academy of Neurology	*www.aan.org*
Association of British Neurologists	*www.theabn.org*
Consortium of MS Centers	*www.mscare.org/cmsc/index.php*
Mellen Center for MS Treatment and Research	*www.clevelandclinic.org/mellen*
National Multiple Sclerosis Society	*www.nmss.org*

Information on clinical trials

US National Institutes of Health	*www.clinicaltrials.gov*
Consortium of MS Centers	*www.mscare.org/cmsc/index.php*
National MS Society	*www.nmss.org*
CenterWatch	*www.centerwatch.com*
TrialX	*www.trialx.com*

American Academy of Neurology grading of evidence used for clinical
recommendations made in this book [1–3]:

> **Class I:** A randomized, controlled trial of the intervention of interest
> with masked or objective outcome assessment, in a representative
> population. Relevant baseline characteristics are presented and sub-
> stantially equivalent among treatment groups or there is appropriate
> statistical adjustment for differences.

J. A. Cohen and A. Rae-Grant, *Handbook of Multiple Sclerosis*,
DOI: 10.1007/978-1-907673-50-4, © Springer Healthcare 2012

Class II: A randomized, controlled clinical trial of the intervention of interest in a representative population with masked or objective assessment that lacks one criterion a–e in Class I or a prospective matched cohort study with masked or objective outcome assessment in a representative population that meets b–e in Class I. Relevant baseline characteristics are presented and substantially equivalent among treatment groups or there is appropriate statistical adjustment for differences.

Class III: All other controlled trials (including well-defined natural history controls or patients serving as their own controls) in a representative population, where outcome is independently assessed, or independently derived by objective outcome measurements.

Class IV: Studies not meeting Class I, II, or III criteria including consensus or expert opinion.

References

1   French J, Gronseth G. Lost in a jungle of evidence: we need a compass. *Neurology.* 2008;71:1634-1638.
2   Gronseth G, French J. Practice parameters and technology assessments: what they are, what they are not, and why you should care. *Neurology.* 2008;71:1639-1643.
3   Gross RA, Johnston KC. Levels of evidence: taking neurology to the next level. *Neurology.* 2008;72:8-10.

Printed by Publishers' Graphics LLC